W0006480

Critical Appraisal from Papers to Patient

A Practical Guide

DUNCAN BOOTLAND • EVAN COUGHLAN
ROBERT GALLOWAY • STEPHANIE GOUBET
EMILY MCWHIRTER

CRC Press
Taylor & Francis Group
Boca Raton London New York

CRC Press is an imprint of the
Taylor & Francis Group, an **informa** business

CRC Press
Taylor & Francis Group
6000 Broken Sound Parkway NW, Suite 300
Boca Raton, FL 33487-2742

Printed and bound by CPI Group (UK) Ltd, Croydon, CR0 4YY
Version Date: 20161010

International Standard Book Number-13: 978-1-4822-3045-1 (Paperback)

Library of Congress Cataloging-in-Publication Data

Names: Bootland, Duncan, author. | Coughlan, Evan, author. | Galloway, Robert, author. | Goubet, Stephanie, author. | McWhirter, Emily, author. | Title: Critical appraisal from papers to patient : a practical guide / Duncan Bootland, Evan Coughlan, Robert Galloway, Stephanie Goubet, and Emily McWhirter. Description: Boca Raton : CRC Press, [2017] | Includes bibliographical references. Identifiers: LCCN 2016026644 (print) | LCCN 2016027455 (ebook) | ISBN 9781482230451 (pbk. : alk. paper) | ISBN 9781482230475 () Subjects: | MESH: Evidence-Based Medicine | Test Taking Skills | Statistics as Topic | Examination Questions Classification: LCC R723.7 (print) | LCC R723.7 (ebook) | NLM WB 18.2 | DDC 616--dc23 LC record available at https://lccn.loc.gov/2016026644

Visit the Taylor & Francis Web site at
http://www.taylorandfrancis.com

and the CRC Press Web site at
http://www.crcpress.com

Contents

Foreword ... vii
Authors ... ix
Introduction ... xi

Section 1 Introduction to Critical Appraisal

1 Types of Papers and Grades of Evidence 3

2 An Approach to Appraising Papers 9

Section 2 Basic Statistics

3 Types of Data and Moving from Samples to Populations 21

4 The Statistics Used in Papers 33

5 Basic Probability 43

Section 3 Appraising Different Types of Papers

6 Observational Studies 55

7 Qualitative Papers 67

8 Therapeutic Papers 73

9 Diagnostic Papers and Screening Papers 91

10 Prognostic Papers 113

11 Economic Studies 119

12 Meta-Analysis 123

Section 4 Applying the Knowledge

13 Writing a Clinical Topic Review 129

14 Running a Journal Club 133

15 Creating a 'Best Available' Evidence-Based Clinical Environment 137

Section 5 Critical Appraisal Exams

16 An Approach to Critical Appraisal Exams 145

17 Practice Papers 153

Glossary 183

Index 197

Foreword

Professor Sir Cyril Chantler, a paediatrician and former chair of the Kings Fund, once told a parliamentary patient safety committee that "Medicine used to be simple, ineffective and relatively safe." Today of course the reverse is true. As it has grown in capability, medicine has also become more complex, expensive and dangerous.

A century ago, medicine was a thing of fine craft, delivered by individuals guided as much by dogma as anything else. The efficacy of interventions was determined largely by the response of individual patients to discrete interventions and an over-valued sense of the causal connection between the two. Today we know better. We understand our treatments and their consequences as a thing of statistical probability.

We improve our outcomes largely through marginal gains, finding our survival advantage in small fractions has spread across large populations. And as a result, for the inhabitants of high-income countries, life has never been safer or longer lived. This is a far better world but, consequently, one in which the efficacy of our interventions is rarely obvious at the end of the bed. In medicine today, the benefits we deliver and the harm we inflict are largely invisible.

In this world we save lives by knowing the evidence offered to us in published research, by not being seduced by poorly or falsely constructed arguments, by designing studies that can tease apart the differences in our outcomes and by understanding the limits of the foundation of knowledge on which we base our decisions.

Today, a working knowledge of statistics and the ability to appraise the medical literature intelligently is as essential to your practice as a knowledge of gross anatomy. This text represents a brilliant primer and the tools and skills it equips the clinician with are designed to help them navigate the uncertainties of medical practice today.

Kevin J. Fong

Authors

Duncan Bootland, MBBS, BSc, FRCEM (@dbootland)
Emergency Medicine Consultant, Brighton and Sussex University Hospitals NHS Trust

Duncan Bootland trained at University College London and has worked in south-east England since then. His specialist training was in Emergency Medicine and Intensive Care, as well as working for Kent, Surrey, Sussex Helicopter Emergency Medicine Service. He was appointed an emergency medicine consultant in 2012. Bootland has an excellent reputation in teaching, especially for the Royal College of Emergency Medicine examinations and in critical appraisal courses.

Evan Coughlan, MB Bch NUI, MRCSEd, DSEM, FRCEM, DipTox (@Evpco)
Emergency Medicine Consultant, Brighton and Sussex University Hospitals NHS Trust

Evan Coughlan qualified in Ireland and finished his registrar training in the United Kingdom. He was appointed as a consultant in 2010. His interests are in ultrasound, trauma and toxicology. He is a passionate and established teacher of critical appraisal courses. He has also written chapters for several textbooks.

Robert Galloway, MBBS, BSc, MRCP, FRCEM, PGCMedED (@drrobgalloway)
Emergency Medicine Consultant, Brighton and Sussex University Hospitals NHS Trust, and Honorary Senior Lecturer and Sub-Dean, Brighton and Sussex Medical School

Robert Galloway trained at St George's Hospital Medical School, London. He dual trained in Emergency Medicine and Intensive Care and was appointed an emergency medicine consultant in 2011. He has a passion for education and has completed a PGC in medical education. He is a Honorary Senior Lecturer, year five sub-dean and leads for Emergency Medicine undergraduate education at Brighton and Sussex Medical School. He has interests in a wide range of academic topics including resuscitation and human factors. He teaches critical appraisal courses with the aim of making them relevant to practicing clinicians.

Stephanie Goubet, MSc
Medical Statistician, Brighton and Sussex University Hospitals NHS Trust and Brighton and Sussex Medical School

Stephanie Goubet came to the Brighton and Sussex University Hospital National Institute for Health Research Clinical Research Facility from the Department of Primary Care and Population Health, University College London. While there she was a member of their Evidence-Based Medicine workshops. She shares her time between Brighton and Sussex University Hospitals NHS Trust and Brighton and Sussex Medical School.

Emily McWhirter, PhD, BSc, RN (@McWhirterEmily)
Director of Performance and Governance, Kent Surrey and Sussex Air Ambulance, and Research Fellow, University of Brighton

Emily McWhirter trained as a nurse at St Thomas' Hospital, London, and later as a midwife at the Nightingale Institute at King's College University. She completed a PhD in 2011 at the University of Brighton to understand the changing role and identity of the contemporary ward manager. Her research interests centre around understanding the connections between the patient experience and clinical outcome.

Introduction

To get from A to B, you only need to know how to drive your car – not how the engine, automatic braking system and gearbox work. If you felt like you had to have this type of understanding, you would not bother driving in the first place.

It is the same when it comes to reading papers; you do not need to understand how they obtained the complex statistical results, but merely what the results and statistics mean, whether they can be trusted and if the study should influence your practice.

Being able to read a journal paper, understand critical appraisal and practice 'best available' evidence-based medicine is a vital skill for all those who work in health care. Integrating this with the knowledge of available skills and resources, along with the patient's preferences, allows us to provide the quality care that our patients deserve.

Evidenced-based medicine (EBM) does not mean that we should only use medical treatments based on high-quality randomized controlled trials (RCTs). That would be madness; there has never been an RCT on whether removing an appendix for appendicitis actually saves lives – we know it does from the best available evidence, in this case, case series. But in order to provide the best possible care for our patients, we need to practice best available EBM, whatever the 'level' that evidence is. In order to do this, we need to understand critical appraisal.

Despite its importance in all fields of medicine, critical appraisal is misunderstood by many, if not most, health care professionals and this is to the detriment of our patients.

Traditionally, math experts who know a lot about how to derive the normal distribution, the math behind chi-squared calculations and how to calculate the exact Yates' correction coefficient have taught critical appraisal and medical statistics. And sometimes confusion is created, not because they do not understand it, but because they understand it too well and do not articulate the clinical relevance and what clinicians need to know.

We think a new approach is needed, hence why we have written this book and started to put on courses in this area. We are not experts; we are clinicians who need a working knowledge of critical appraisal in order to appropriately influence our practice. We know what is needed to read a journal article, understand the results, whether to believe the results and whether we should implement the results with our patients.

When it comes to p-values, confidence intervals and normal distributions, we do not know the formulas to derive them, but we know their importance and how to interpret the results. And that is a good thing because it is all you need to know when reading a paper as a clinician.

We want this book to take you on a journey: from frightened by the thought of a confidence interval, and so never looking at a journal article, to being able to enjoy reading and understanding articles (and not just the abstracts) speedily, while deciding whether they will change your practice.

We will not be teaching you how the engine and gearbox of critical appraisal work, merely how to drive. That is all you need, and that is all you want. After reading this book, you will be able to trust your own assessment of papers and not be influenced by the sandwiches and cheap pens of reps, however alluring their smile.

The book takes a stepwise approach to critical appraisal, starting with why we need to bother with critical appraisal, moving to the types of papers and research you may encounter, and ending with how to dissect the papers.

Throughout the book, the main text contains the essential information, with 'Nerd's Corner' boxes for those who are interested and want to get a deeper understanding. There is also a Glossary of Terms for easy reference and revision.

For those who have critical appraisal exams coming up, there is guidance on how to approach and pass these, including practice papers.

We hope you enjoy this textbook as well as find it a valuable resource for passing exams, writing essays and, most importantly, treating patients in the best possible way.

For further information on our associated courses, please go to the website www.medicalcriticalappraisal.com.

Thanks for reading.

Section 1

Introduction to Critical Appraisal

1 Types of Papers and Grades of Evidence

It is nearing the end of a Friday evening in the medical assessment unit, and lying on the trolley in front of me is a 47-year-old man who has attended complaining of breathlessness and a sharp left-sided chest pain. I am tired and want to go home, but even as a consultant, I am made anxious by the knowledge that chest pain is one of the 'banana skins' of our profession.

As much as any other, this situation reflects the challenges we face many times a day: What clinical information do I need to glean from my history and examination? What clinical decision tools should I use? What diagnostic tests should I subject my patient to and how confident can I be in them? When I finally make the diagnosis, what is the best treatment?

The ability to interpret the evidence and the guidelines that already exist and the new ones that are published every month, and to do this in a way that leaves enough time to actually see some patients, is challenging. We need to remember that our desire to know how to treat our patients better should drive our aim to understand evidence-based medicine (EBM), and then an understanding of EBM should drive improvements in patient care.

Before we begin trying to work out how to dissect various papers, we need to understand how research is divided into different types, and which types are best for answering which questions.

TYPES OF PAPERS

Reading through the medical literature, it will not take you long to realize that there are a number of different types of studies out there – the EBM world is not just randomized controlled trials (RCTs), diagnostic studies and meta-analyses.

The way different study types are grouped together depends in some part on whom you speak to, but we find the following to be useful in ordering our thoughts when it comes to the different types. Think about three questions:

1. What sort of environment (a clinical laboratory, a highly controlled but still clinical setting, a normal ward or general practitioner's surgery, etc.) is the trial being performed in?
2. What sort of results are the researchers interested in? Is it a result like mortality rate or blood pressure which will provide a numerical value, or is it a subjective feeling or description of outcomes and emotions which cannot be reduced to a numerical value (qualitative research)?

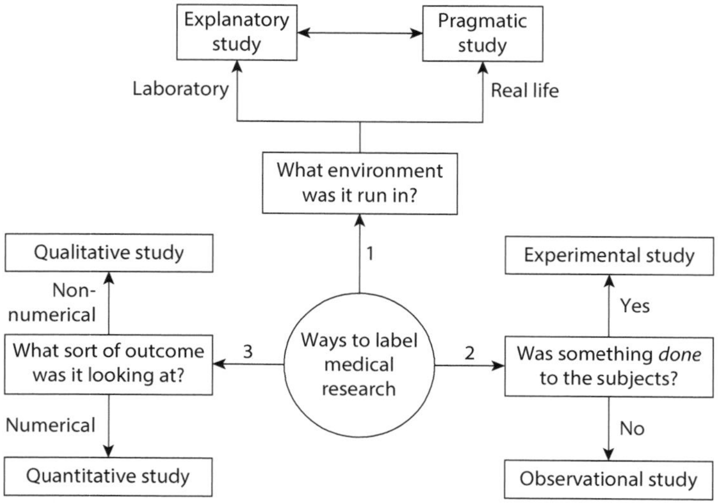

FIGURE 1.1 Different ways to label a trial – three questions to ask.

3. Are the researchers planning to do something to the patient, for example, give them a new drug or do a new diagnostic test, or are they just observing what happens to them?

The answers to these three questions should then allow us to describe the trial as explanatory or pragmatic, qualitative or quantitative and experimental or observational (Figure 1.1). Remember that these labels are not exclusive, and so it is possible to have, for example, a pragmatic, qualitative, experimental trial. The labels simply allow us to begin to order our thoughts about what has gone on within the trial.

Question 1: What Sort of Environment Was the Trial Run In?

As a rough rule clinical trials can be run in two sorts of places: highly controlled settings such as research laboratories (often with carefully selected, specific patients) or actual clinical settings that are more prone to the normal variations in atmosphere, patients, time of the day and staffing levels. Explanatory research is conducted in the more highly controlled environment and gives the best chance of seeing if the intervention actually works if as many as possible outside influencing factors are taken out of the equation. Pragmatic research, however, is performed in a setting more like a clinical environment (or actually *in* a clinical environment) and gives a better idea of whether the intervention will work in the real world. Clearly there are a variety of settings in which, and patient types on whom, studies can be performed. It is wise to consider the type of study as being on a spectrum between the explanatory and pragmatic; the more tightly controlled the conditions of the study, the closer to being explanatory and vice versa.

Question 2: What Sort of Results Are the Researchers Interested In?

Whether the result that is generated is a hard clinical number such as blood pressure, height or mortality rate or is instead something less quantifiable like sense of well-being or happiness is our second way of dividing up research. Quantitative research will generate numbers such as difference in blood pressure or mortality, which can then be analyzed to produce the statistical results that we talk about later in the book and which form much of the published results from medical literature. Studies that produce a result given as a description which cannot be boiled down to numerical data (such as opinions, explanations of styles of working and why people do not follow best practice, emotional well-being or thoughts and feelings) are termed qualitative research and can be harder to succinctly analyze and summarize. However, there are established ways of looking at this type of paper to ensure that it is as rigorously conducted as quantitative research. See chapter 7 for information on this increasingly important subject. However, in many studies looking at what you might think of as qualitative outcomes (quality of life being a good example), scoring systems have been developed so that a quantitative result can be recorded (and hence analyzed in a statistically clearer way).

Question 3: Are the Researchers Planning to Do Something to the Patient?

The final way for us to define the type of research is by whether the researchers intervene in the patients' care in any way. In RCTs and in diagnostic studies (both of which we talk about in detail later), but also in other types of study, we take a group of subjects or patients and apply a new treatment, intervention or diagnostic test to their care. These sorts of studies are termed experimental studies. Studies where the researchers look at what happens to a group of subjects or patients but the care that they receive is influenced only by normal practice (and normal variations in practice) and not by the researchers are called observational studies. Surveys, case reports, cohort studies, case control studies and cross-sectional studies are all observational studies, whereas RCTs and diagnostic studies are both experimental studies.

There are a number of different kinds of each type of study, whether experimental/observational, pragmatic/explanatory or qualitative/quantitative. A description of the main features of the important types of studies can be found in the Glossary, and an overview is given in Tables 1.1 and 1.2. The type of study that the researchers perform should be decided before they start and should be based on the strengths and weaknesses of each type of possible study.

Finally, we need to mention secondary research. Although single papers can be highly valuable, often greater value can be derived from combining the results or knowledge from a number of papers. Results of different studies can be brought together in review articles, systematic reviews or meta-analyses, all of which we discuss later in the book.

TABLE 1.1
Different Types of Experimental Studies

Randomized controlled study (RCT)	The study group is divided into two or more groups by a randomization process. One group is given one intervention, and the other group(s) another. The outcomes in the different groups are then compared. The randomization works to balance and thereby remove the influence of confounding factors. The RCT is considered to be the best sort of experimental study and commonly used in many examinations. They are, however, normally expensive to run.
Diagnostic study	The diagnostic test is performed on the whole study group alongside the gold standard test. The performance of the diagnostic test under investigation is then compared with the gold standard test. Diagnostic studies appear less commonly than RCTs in the literature but appear commonly in many examinations.
Crossover study	The study is designed to compare two interventions (usually drugs). Instead of one group receiving one drug and the other group the second drug, both groups receive one drug for a period of time, followed by the alternate drug for a period of time. The difference between the two groups is the order in which they receive the two drugs. Essentially, each patient is acting as their own control. Importantly, the drugs being studied must not interfere with the process of the underlying disease and the disease must be unlikely to alter in nature during the time course of the trial.
Cluster study	This is another form of trial that compares two or more interventions. Instead of individual patients being randomized to the different arms of the study, groups of patients are randomized. An example is all emergency department (ED) patients from one hospital being randomized to having tea and coffee provided free of charge in the waiting area, and all ED patients in another hospital not receiving that intervention.

GRADES OF EVIDENCE

The main aim of the EBM is to deliver study results that further our understanding about how to diagnose and treat patients. As thousands of studies are published every week, we need a way to judge both the importance of the results and the strength we should ascribe to the recommendations given in the paper's conclusion (or indeed to any guideline produced by an august professional body). Although there are variations in how different people rate different types of study and how strongly they make their recommendations, most follow a similar pattern to that shown in Tables 1.3 and 1.4.

Often people find the ranking of evidence and recommendations a little confusing. Although it is fairly standard that an RCT is considered of more value than a cohort study, and the grading system reflects that, remember it is only a tool to help us when summarizing the evidence that we are reading. To give one famous example, the British Doctors Study was a cohort study performed in the 1950s that

TABLE 1.2
Different Types of Observational Studies

Case control studies	A group of patients with an outcome variable (like the presence of a particular disease) are compared with a group without that outcome. The medical and social histories of both groups can be compared to look for preceding risk factors that may have made the patients with the outcome more susceptible. Case control studies are by definition retrospective and therefore suffer from recall bias. They are good for looking at patients with rare diseases. They are not very good at looking at exposures to rare risk factors.
Cohort study	A group of patients with an exposure to an intervention or risk factor are followed in time and compared with those without the exposure to that intervention or risk factor. The researchers do not alter what exposure any patient gets, and the variation between the two groups is just due to normal differences in care or exposure. The outcomes of both groups are then compared. Although these are normally prospective, if a large database of patients has been created for something else, the database can be used retrospectively to perform cohort studies. Cohort studies are valuable as they allow us to look at a number of different outcomes in relation to one exposure and the time sequence of events can be assessed. Problems include being potentially costly to run and that you need a large sample size if you want to look at rare outcomes.
Cross-sectional studies	Disease and exposure status of a population are studied at the same time. They are good for establishing prevalence or association. Unfortunately, a large number of subjects is normally needed, and they cannot be used to demonstrate causation.

TABLE 1.3
Ranking the Types of Study

Grade	Type of Paper
1	Systematic review (including at least one RCT) or a single good-quality RCT
2	Studies without randomization
3	Well-designed, controlled observational studies such as cohort studies or case control studies
4	Observational studies such as case series or case reports
5	Expert opinion

TABLE 1.4
Ranking the Strength of the Recommendation Made from the EBM Available

Grade	Usual Basis for Strength of Recommendation
A	Based on meta-analyses, systematic reviews or randomized controlled trial
B	Based on level 2 or 3 evidence (see above)
C	Based on level 4 evidence
D	Based on expert advice

proved to be a major factor in demonstrating the link between smoking and lung cancer. If you applied Tables 1.3 and 1.4 literally, it would only be considered level 3 evidence and a grade B recommendation not to smoke. From this example you can see that there are situations where an RCT is neither the best nor only way to provide a world-changing result.

Take-Home Message

1. Studies can be described as explanatory or pragmatic depending on whether the trial was run in highly controlled conditions or real-life conditions, experimental or observational depending on whether the researchers intervene in the care of the patients, and qualitative or quantitative depending on whether the results are the patients' descriptions of feelings or numerical data.
2. There are a number of different study designs for both observational and experimental studies, and which ones the researchers choose will depend on what they are studying and the type of result they are looking for.
3. The different types of papers are graded by how valuable within the EBM world they are, with meta-analyses and RCTs at the top.
4. The strength of recommendation that is made by groups such as the National Institute for Health and Care Excellence (NICE) or Royal Colleges based on the available EBM is usually also graded, with recommendations made on the basis of results from meta-analyses and RCTs considered the strongest.

2 An Approach to Appraising Papers

A very simple approach when reading papers is to think about the following questions:

1. Is the question they are trying to answer relevant to your practice and patients?
2. Are the results significant (clinically and statistically) and if so, should this affect how I treat my patients?
3. Is it of high enough quality that I can trust this paper (internal validity)?
4. Is it relevant to the patients whom I see (external validity)?
5. If the answer to all of these is yes (and the side effects of the treatment/diagnostic test are acceptable), then how do we implement the findings?

With this is mind, you can now think about dissecting individual papers. Papers are not single units; they consist of multiple parts. In this chapter, we look at what these parts are. This chapter refers predominantly to interventional trials, but other papers follow a similar approach. The specific details of how to assess each type of paper are given in the specific chapters.

The purpose of research is to answer a clinical question, which we all meet in our day-to-day clinical practice. For example, in a patient with a wrist fracture, we might ask ourselves a number of questions: Which is better to make the diagnosis, x-ray or ultrasound (diagnostic study)? Is a haematoma block or Bier's block a better anaesthetic (therapeutic study)? To answer this we would need to perform a literature review, and if we find there is insufficient evidence to choose one over the other, it may prompt us to do a study.

In a study, we enrol a sufficient quantity of patients, and once we have the raw data we use statistics to present the evidence and decide whether one is better than the other. We can then answer our question in light of our results plus any previous research. We are now in a position to write our paper and submit it for publication.

Prior to 1993, the way in which studies were written for publications varied tremendously. The Consolidated Standards of Reporting Trials (CONSORT) statement has meant that randomized controlled trials (RCTs) should now be reported in a specific way. A full description of the CONSORT statement is available online at http://www.consort-statement.org. This systematic way of presenting studies is aimed at therapeutic studies; however, it is equally valid for diagnostic papers and observational studies.

Putting it into the simplest terms, papers can be divided into the following sections:

- Title: Quick-to-read explanation of what is being studied
- Abstract: Short summary of the whole paper

- Introduction: States the clinical question and a summary of the findings of the authors' literature review
- Methods: Explains how the study has been designed
- Results: Shows the number of patients enrolled, those who dropped out and what the researchers' findings were
- Discussion and conclusions: Explains the results in the setting of previous research and answers the clinical question

Now, let's discuss these sections in more detail.

TITLE

The first thing we notice on picking up any paper is the title. The title is often used to sieve papers when performing a literature review and as such is important. The title should be clear and give us an idea of what clinical question is being studied. It may also give an indication of the study design.

ABSTRACT

An abstract is a summary of the whole paper, usually set out in the same way as the main text. It allows the reader to get a feel for what was done, what results were found and what conclusions were drawn by the authors, but it will not allow the reader sufficient detail to properly appraise the paper. It does, however, allow a second level of sieving of papers when performing a literature review.

INTRODUCTION

The introduction should state the research question the authors have designed the paper to answer. It should describe the importance of the clinical question, what is already known about the clinical question and why further study is necessary. *The research question can usually be found in the last paragraph of the introduction.* Once we know this information, we can decide if we think that the clinical question is important and relevant to our practice.

At this point in reading the paper, it is valuable to think about how *you* would have designed a study to answer the question the authors have set themselves. As you read through the methods, compare the design that the authors have chosen to the one you would have chosen.

METHODS

The methods section describes the design of the study and how it was subsequently run. There may be an ideal study design, but this may not be practical for many reasons, such as finances, ethics or availability of patients. The study design takes these practicalities into account, but in reality, trials do not always run to the protocol they were designed to follow.

The elements that should appear in the methods section of a trial can be remembered by the acronym PICOT:

P – Population
I – Intervention
C – Comparison
O – Outcome measures
T – Time

Population

The first thing to check in assessing the methodology of a study is the population being studied.

- How did the authors pick their study population?
- Where was it set: in a GP (General Practice) surgery, in an outpatient clinic or somewhere else?
- Is the study population representative of the population that we are interested in? That is, if we are working in emergency medicine, was the study done on patients who present to emergency departments?

Now consider who was included and who was excluded:

- What were the inclusion criteria?
- Did they include all the patients we would have included?
- What were the exclusion criteria?
- Were any groups of patients excluded that should not have been?

Having too strict inclusion and exclusion criteria may lead to an experimental group that is no longer representative of the population as a whole. This is known as diagnostic purity bias.

Next, think about the sample size in the study:

- How did the authors come to this sample size?
- Did they calculate it using a sample size calculation and if so, did they quote all the factors required for this calculation?

In many diagnostic or observational studies, the sample size calculation is not mentioned in the paper; however, it should be.

Finally, we consider how we draw our sample from the general population.

- What type of sampling did the authors use?

When taking a sample, we want it to represent the population in which we are interested (Figure 2.1). There are many different methods of taking a sample.

- *Random sampling* is where patients are randomly taken from the population in which you are interested.

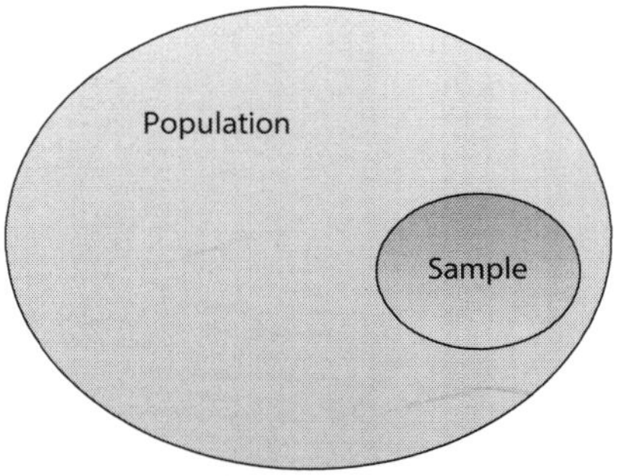

FIGURE 2.1 Sample size with respect to population.

- *Systematic sampling* is where every *n*th patient is chosen (*n*th can be any number, e.g. every third or every fourth).
- *Stratified sampling* involves taking a random sample from different strata of a population, for example, a random sample from smokers and non-smokers. Generally, the best method is for the numbers in each sample group to reflect the size of each of these groups in the general population. For example, if 30% of the population were smokers and we were to sample 100 people, then 30 people would be enrolled who are smokers. Stratified sampling may allow for a smaller sample size to be used and hence can be more cost-effective. It provides for a more representative sample and can allow better inferences to be made about specific subgroups.
- *Cluster sampling* is where instead of enrolling individual patients, we enrol groups of patients. Imagine we were looking at the impact of *bare below the elbows*. We could look at 10 hospitals where we compare bare below the elbow and 10 where we do not. We would have enrolled the hospitals, not the individual patients. Cluster sampling can be used when sampling of individuals is difficult or impossible. A regular example of this is in papers examining changes in service delivery. However, cluster sampling may not reflect the diversity of the population as a whole and sampling errors are more common. If you take a random sample of clusters, it is a one-stage cluster sampling; if you also take a random sample within each cluster as well as a random sample of clusters, this is known as a two-stage cluster sampling.
- *Convenience sampling* is a sample taken when it is convenient for the researchers of the study, for example, enrolling patients during office hours. This method of sampling is quick and easy but is prone to bias as the sample is likely not to be representative of the whole population.
- *Consecutive sampling* is similar to convenience sampling, but with this form of sampling we try to enrol every patient who is available to us.

Fundamentally, we need to know whether the sample is representative of the population the authors wanted to study and of the population we are interested in.

Intervention and Comparison

In therapeutic studies, those enrolled undergo some form of intervention, which is compared with current practice or another treatment. In diagnostic studies we compare a test with a gold standard. In observational studies we look to compare the effects of different exposures which exist between different populations but which we did not intervene to create.

- What is the intervention in the study? What treatment, exposure or diagnostic test is being looked at?
- What is the comparison? In a therapeutic trial, what is the control, and in a diagnostic study, what is the gold standard?
- What are the baseline characteristics of the patients, and in therapeutic trials are they the same between these two groups?
    - Generally, 'Table 1' in the paper gives a list of patient baseline characteristics, and it is always worth looking at this to make sure that there are no obvious differences between the groups.
- Have the authors identified any confounding factors? If so, how have they been taken into account?
- If none have been identified, are there any confounders that should have been taken into account?

There are specific questions to ask for therapeutic, observational or diagnostic studies that are covered later. Do not worry if you are unsure of some of the concepts mentioned here, as we cover them in later chapters.

Outcome Measures

The type of outcome we look at depends on whether it is a diagnostic or therapeutic or observational trial. In therapeutic papers we need to ask:

- What are the outcome measures?
- What is the primary outcome measure?
- Is this appropriate?
    - Outcome measures should be reliable (they should give the same result each time a measurement is performed if there has been no change), valid (how well they measure what we are expecting them to measure) and responsive (able to detect a change).
- Is the outcome measure clinically relevant, such as mortality, or is a surrogate end point used?
    - A surrogate end point is an outcome measure that is used instead of a clinically relevant one, usually because it allows the trial to be smaller and to take less time. It also allows studies to be performed that would otherwise not be possible due to cost or an inability to enrol enough patients, for example, using gastric pH instead of the rate of GI bleeding when looking at proton pump inhibitors.

In diagnostic studies, the outcome measure is a measure of the ability of the test under investigation to diagnose the disease.

Time

It is important to assess if adequate time has been allotted to enrol and follow up patients.

- How long did it take to enrol the required number of subjects?
    - Taking a long time to enrol might suggest that the inclusion and exclusion criteria were too restrictive.
- Were patients followed up and if so, for how long and was this length of time appropriate?
    - Ideally, patients should be followed up for an adequate period to determine whether they return to full function or have any complications of the treatment.
- Were there many dropouts and if so, why did they drop out?
    - It is not unusual for patients to drop out of a study or be lost to follow-up. However, if this number is large, it may be because of treatment side effects or a difficult-to-tolerate regimen, which may limit the treatment's usefulness. The authors should explain why patients dropped out so we can assess this.

RESULTS

The results section of the paper tells the findings of the study. It should tell how many patients were enrolled and how many patients dropped out or were lost to follow-up. We must consider:

- Did the authors enrol the required sample size?
- How many patients were excluded?
- How many patients dropped out or were lost to follow-up?
- Were all the patients compliant with the study protocol?
- Is the number of patients who dropped out of the study similar to the number estimated by the authors when they performed their sample size calculation?
- What was the number of protocol violations?
- Did the authors take into account dropouts and protocol violations in their analysis?
- Is there a CONSORT flow diagram or similar table for explanation of recruitment?
- Have the authors reported the appropriate statistics?
    - For therapeutic and many observational trials, the authors should mention relative risk, absolute risk reduction, relative risk reduction and number needed to treat. For diagnostic studies they should quote sensitivity, specificity and ideally likelihood ratios and predictive values.

The authors should present their results in a way that can be easily understood by the reader. You should be able to draw a contingency (2 × 2) table from the data and ensure that the authors correctly quoted statistics. You might think that the quoted statistics are never wrong, but it can happen.

DISCUSSION AND CONCLUSIONS

The discussion should critically look at the study, outline how the results of the study fit into the current literature and explain how the authors have come to the conclusion they have. It should give us the limitations of the study and explain any ways in which the authors tried to take these into account. When reading the discussion and conclusion section consider:

- Are the results a surprise or expected?
- Why do the authors think this is?
- What limitations do the authors give?
- Are there any other limitations the authors have not mentioned?
- Are their conclusions valid?
- Do they match your own conclusions?

At this point it is important to consider the validity of the study. There are two types of validity: *internal validity* and *external validity*. Internal validity is our assessment of the methodology of the study and whether this permits us to believe the results from this sample of patients. External validity is the extent to which the study can be extrapolated to the wider population beyond this sample of patients and in particular to our own local population.

After having decided about internal and external validity, the next thing to decide is whether the result of the study is important for your patients. If it is, then consider implementing it. This is not as easy as it sounds; there are many barriers which may prevent implementation of the intervention. We remember this as the 4 Bs:

- *Badness*: What harms are caused by the intervention?
- *Burden of disease*: Is it so rare that no one cares?
- *Budget*: Can we afford to make the changes?
- *Beliefs*: How will we educate people about this new intervention, and how will we deal with intransigent colleagues?

OTHER FACTORS TO CONSIDER

BIAS

Bias is a systematic error in the way observations were made, or the experiment is carried out, which leads to inaccuracy. Many types of bias have been described. Figure 2.2 and Table 2.1 give a list of the most common types of bias. Although we have listed a number of types of bias for information, it is more important to understand that bias leads to inaccuracy and how bias occurs rather than knowing the name of each type of bias.

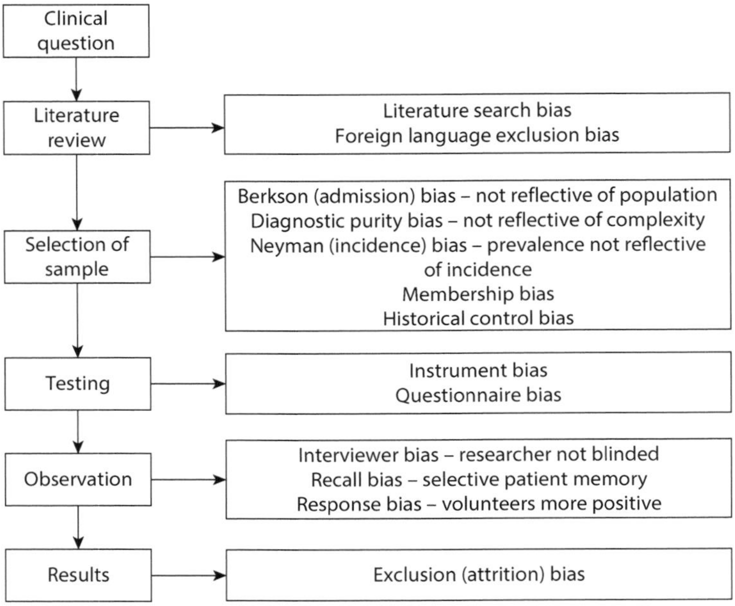

FIGURE 2.2 Types of bias from each stage of a study.

Bias can be combated by means of:

- A comprehensive literature review
- Consecutive patient enrolment
- Prospective study design – designing the study before you collect data
- Randomization
- Concealed allocation
- Blinding
- Use of intention-to-treat analysis

Authors and Institution

The list of authors of the paper is given a highly prominent and therefore important place in the write-up of any study. We need to be aware of the potential for our opinion about a paper to be influenced by the person or people who have written it. There are certain authors whose papers we are more likely to read and whose conclusions we are more likely to believe. This is particularly true of those authors who have a research pedigree. It *is* reasonable for us to consider that studies performed by these people are likely to be of good quality, but we must never lose sight of the fact that each paper must be judged on its individual merits.

It is also worth taking note of the institution or institutions in which the study was performed. Some institutions, like some authors, will be renowned for high-quality research, but remember that the environment in which the study is run impacts heavily on its external validity.

TABLE 2.1
Types of Bias

Type of Bias	Type of Study	Explanation
Attrition	Therapeutic	Loss of subjects in a study leading to inequality between the two groups with respect to exposure and/or outcome.
Berkson	Case control	Patients who present to hospital may not be representative of community as a whole.
Diagnostic purity	Therapeutic	Exclusion criteria are too tight and so the study group may not be representative of the complexity of disease in the community.
Foreign language	Systematic review and meta-analysis	Less likely to include studies not published in English in a literature review.
Historical control	Observational	Apart from the intervention being studied, there may be a difference in management and prognosis between the research group and the controls simply because medical care improves (or should improve) over time.
Interviewer	Observational	The interviewer's opinions, prejudices and even non-verbal cues may influence the responses of subjects.
Language	Meta-analysis	English language papers are more likely to be published.
Literature search	Meta-analysis	Studies are more likely to be used if from a journal with a better reputation in a literature review.
Measurement	Diagnostic	Inaccurate measurement tool used.
Membership	Therapeutic	People who choose to be members of a group may differ in important respects to the general community.
Multiple publication	Meta-analysis	Variations of the same research or even the same study published in different journals.
Neyman	Observational	A bias seen in observational studies where we look at the links between a risk factor and the chance of getting acertain disease. If that disease causes the death of patients and our study only looks at survivors at any one point, we may underestimate the effect of the risk factor.
Non-respondent	Observational	Responders may differ significantly from non-responders.
Publication	Meta-analysis	Positive results are more likely to be published.
Questionnaire	Observational	Questions may be written to lead the respondent towards a particular reply.
Recall	Observational	Subjects with the disease are more likely to remember a potential causative agent than controls.
Response	Observational	Subjects may shape their response in order to please the interviewer.

Financial Interests

We have mentioned that studies cost money to run. Ask yourself:

- Where did the money come from for the study?
- Did the authors have any financial interest in the results of the study?

References

The last section of the paper is the reference section. You might question the use of a list of studies. In fact, the reference section is often a gold mine of information. When reading the paper look through the reference list to see what foundation the authors have built their study upon and to check whether you think they have missed any significant papers from the literature. Assess whether the number of references given, and the papers that the authors have drawn them from, represent a reasonable evidence base for the study performed.

Publishing Journal

A final point to note is in which journal the paper has been published. In the same way as considering who the authors are, we need to remember to not be too influenced by what journal a paper is published in, but to be aware that the larger journals have a bigger reviewing staff and in-house statisticians to check the internal validity of a trial before it is published. Because of this, most people feel instinctively more confident in the results of papers published in the bigger journals.

Many journals have an impact factor associated with them. The impact factor of a journal reflects how widely the papers it publishes are cited in the medical literature and as such can be seen as a measure of how important or 'big' a journal is.

Take-Home Message

1. A study consists of many parts and these can be divided into title, abstract, introduction, methods, results, discussion and conclusions.
2. The methods section can be divided into PICOT (population, intervention, comparison, outcome measures and time).
3. When reading a paper, consider the factors that are affecting internal validity and the factors that are affecting external validity.
4. There are many forms of bias – knowledge of each individual type is not necessary but understanding the concept is.

Section 2

Basic Statistics

3 Types of Data and Moving from Samples to Populations

An in-depth knowledge of statistics is not needed for you to be able to read a paper and decide if you think it is any good. However, to be able to justify your opinion and to be sure that you are not rejecting or accepting the paper's conclusions incorrectly, a basic grounding in general statistics *is* needed and, over the next three chapters, we endeavour to give you that. In some cases we expand beyond what we feel is core, which will be covered in 'Nerd's Corner' rather than in the main text. This information will add to your understanding of the subject as a whole and so is valuable, but do not worry if you struggle with it or do not want to commit it to memory. If you do not feel up to 'Nerd's Corner' at all, you are quite welcome to move on to the next part in the main text. In this chapter we cover three main concepts: types of data, ways to describe the data including types of distribution and measures of spread, and using sample data to make inferences about whole populations.

TYPES OF DATA

The aim of most studies is to collect data from investigations performed on a sample of the population and then analyze that data to come to a conclusion about the population. Obviously, the type of data that is collected during a study will vary depending on what is being studied – for example, when you are looking at hair colour, the results you get are fundamentally and instinctively different from the type of result you get when looking at weight or height. From a critical appraisal point of view, this is important because the way in which data about hair colour is analyzed requires different statistical tests than data about weight or height. In-depth knowledge about what statistical tests are done is not essential (although we mention this later in a 'Nerd's Corner'), but knowledge about how different data is described is needed. We find the flow chart in Figure 3.1 to be the easiest and best way to demonstrate the different ways to describe groups of data.

Quantitative data is where a numerical value can be given to the data and this can be either discrete (e.g. with the number of people in a club, it can be 3 or 4 but not 3.5) or continuous, where it can be anywhere on a scale. Categorical data (also called qualitative data) is where there is a fixed number of defined categories into which data is organized and this can be either nominal (i.e. given a name), such as hair

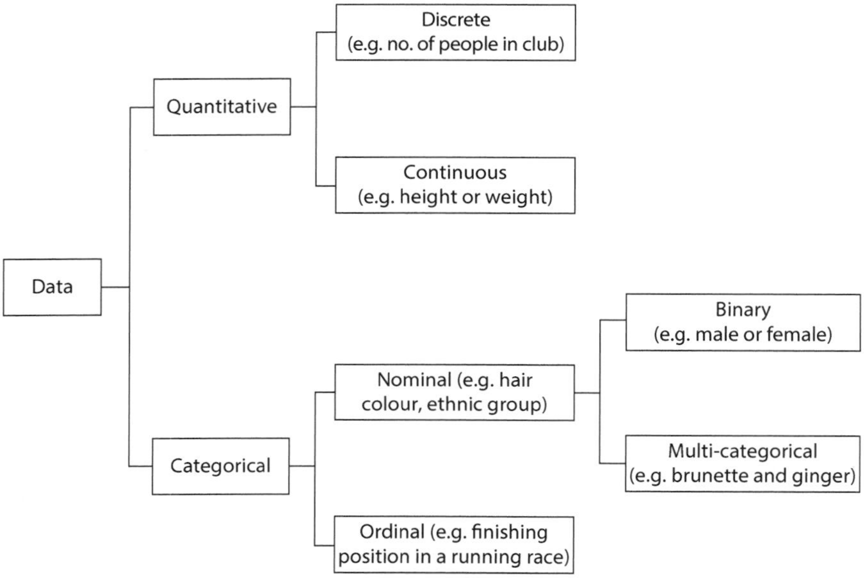

FIGURE 3.1 The main types of data.

colour, or ordinal (i.e. where there is a rank to the categories), such as first, second and third place in a race.

For completeness and while we are talking about data it seems reasonable to add a description of the accepted definitions of various types of epidemiological data (Table 3.1). As ever, we would strongly recommend that an understanding of what each term means rather than rote learning of a definition is the most valuable approach.

TABLE 3.1
Epidemiological Data

Term	Explanation
Incidence	The rate that new cases appear over a period of time divided by the population size
Standardized (mortality) rate	The (mortality) rate where an adjustment has been made to compensate for confounding factors
Point prevalence	The number of people with the disease at a given point in time divided by the size of the population at that time
Period prevalence	The number of people with the disease in a period of time divided by the size of the population during this period
Lifetime prevalence	The proportion of a population that either has or has had the disease up to the point of the study

DESCRIBING THE DATA: QUANTITATIVE DATA

A mass of values collected as part of a study need to be summarized or described in a way that the reader can easily understand and use. It is pointless to simply list each individual value and expect the reader to interpret what it all means – most of us need the help of the author and a statistician to make heads or tails of it all. To help explain the data, there are various things that may be done, including calculating an average, describing how the data are distributed and describing the spread of the data.

Describing the Average Value

An average is a single value that incorporates all the values and so can be helpful in representing the data set in a quick and simple way (Table 3.2).

Describing the Distribution of the Data

If we were to plot all the data from our study on a graph, it might fall into one of a number of shapes, called distributions. Knowledge of distributions is important because it affects which average we use (mean or median) and which measure of spread (inter-quartile range or standard deviation). It also influences what statistical tests we can do on the data.

A number of names are given to various patterns of distribution, but of all the ways that data can be distributed, the ones you must know are the last three shown in Figure 3.2.

Normal Distribution

Figure 3.3 is without doubt the most important type of distribution and is referred to as 'normal', 'bell-shaped' or 'Gaussian'. Due to its fundamental importance in medical statistics and its value to us, we will spend some time discussing it before

TABLE 3.2
Averages

Type of Average	Description	Advantages	Disadvantages
Mean	The sum of all the observations divided by the number of observations	Easy to calculate and understand	Influenced by outliers so less useful with skewed data
Median	The middle number of the group when they are ranked in order; the mean of the two middle values is taken if there is an even number of values	Reduces the effect of outliers and so is useful in skewed data	Exact 95% confidence intervals of the median require specialist knowledge and software to calculate
Mode	The most frequently occurring value in a list	Can be used with categorical data	Less intuitively useful

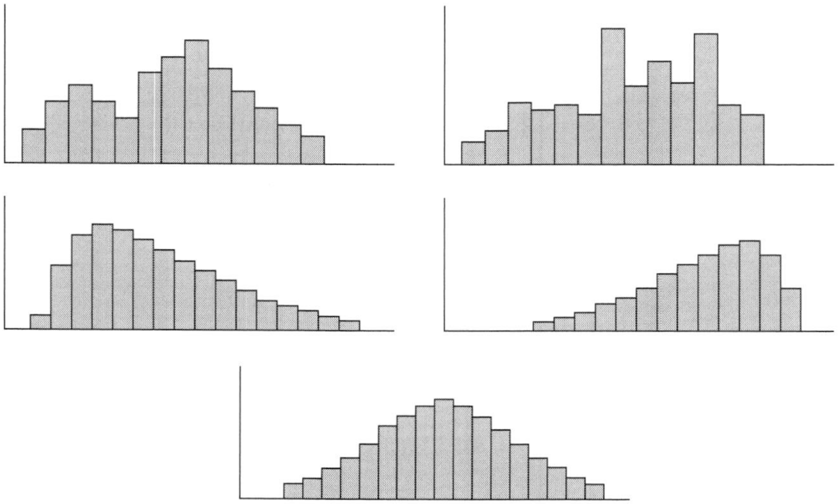

FIGURE 3.2 Various types of distribution.

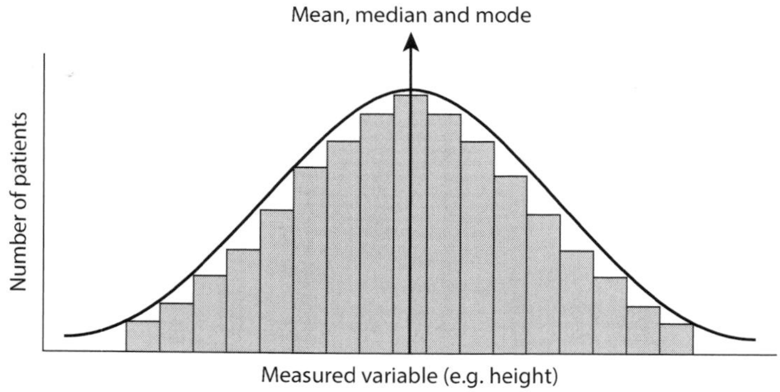

FIGURE 3.3 Normal distribution.

moving on briefly to the two other types of distribution you should be aware of. A normal distribution has a number of important mathematical characteristics, the first of which is that the mean, median and mode all lie at the same point.

Having a data set that is normally distributed allows certain types of statistical tests to be performed on the data, such as t-tests and analysis of variance. These are called parametric tests and they are preferred over non-parametric because they are more robust, or powerful (meaning you need less people in the study). The decision about whether data are actually normally distributed can be done visually by plotting the data on a chart and checking to see if it looks like a bell curve. In small studies this can be unreliable, but one can quickly see whether the data are symmetrical by checking if the mean is equal to the median. There are more formal ways to confirm the normality of your data set, but they are beyond the scope of this book. What is interesting is that the importance of having normally distributed data is such that when faced with a data set that is not normally distributed, many authors will convert their data to a normal distribution through mathematical manipulation so that it can be analyzed with parametric statistical tests.

There are two further important features of normal distributions that allow us to estimate what result we would get in the whole population, based on the results we obtain from a single sample. We discuss these in the next section.

Skewed Data

Normally distributed data will be symmetrically distributed about the middle (remember, mean = median = mode). Some data sets may instead have their values more biased to the left or right of the graph. These are described as skewed data sets and the long tail of the graph indicates whether the data is skewed to the right (positive) (Figure 3.4a) or to the left (negative) (Figure 3.4b). Unlike normally distributed data, the mean, mode and median do not lie at the same point, and this is why we often decide that the mean is not the most appropriate average to use when talking about skewed data.

It is more powerful to analyze normally distributed data than skewed data, and analysts will transform their skewed data into a normal distribution using mathematical tools such as logarithmic transformation.

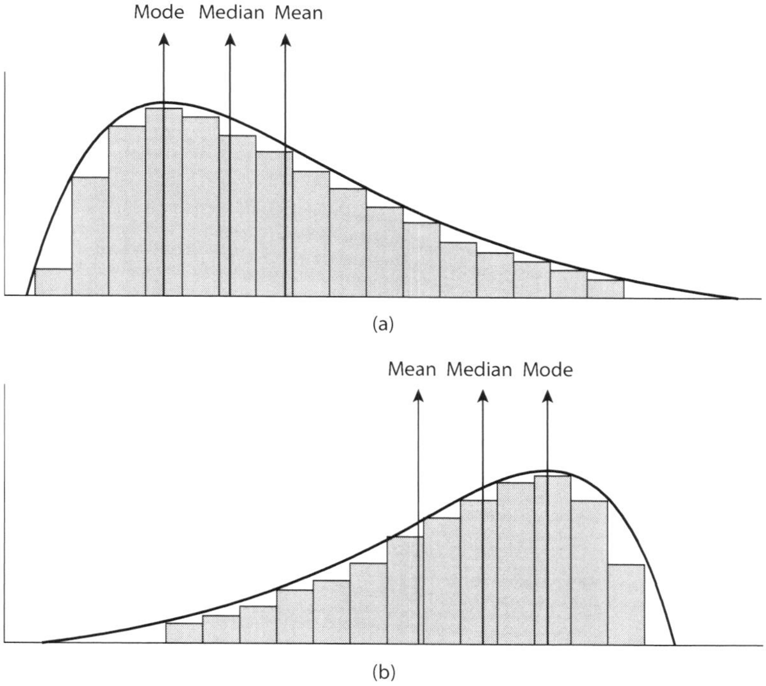

FIGURE 3.4 Skewed data. (a) Right (positive) skewed. (b) Left (negative) skewed.

TABLE 3.3
Measures of Spread and Location for Normal (or Symmetric) and Skewed Data

Distribution	Measure of Spread	Explanation	Average Used
Normal or symmetric	Standard deviation	A value to describe the average variation of each value in a data set from the mean of that set	Mean
Skewed	Inter-quartile range (IQR)	The range between the bottom quarter and the upper quarter of the data set; it is therefore the range of the middle 50% of the data set	Median

Descriptions of How Spread Out the Data Is

As we have seen, the shape of the spread of the data is important to us, but so is how spread out the data is. An average, on its own, does not give sufficient information to get a real feel for the data set, and so an average should be combined with a 'measure of spread' to allow a better understanding of the data. Which measure of spread and average to use depends on how the data is distributed, that is, whether data is normally distributed or skewed (Table 3.3).

The importance of looking at the spread or variance of a pair of samples is that when we try to judge whether there is a genuine difference between the two groups, variance is one of the three factors that we must consider. The other two are sample size and the actual difference between the mean of the two groups. We return to this point when we talk about the power of a study in later chapters.

An inquisitive reader might now ask for more information about standard deviations, and this is given in 'Nerd's Corner'. Remember that you do not necessarily need to learn what is in the 'Nerd's Corner', but an appreciation of the points will help your overall understanding. For those who really struggle with the math, all you really need to know at the moment is that standard deviation is a measure of the spread of the data and it can be calculated from the data set.

Nerd's Corner: Descriptions of the Variance of the Data

Consider two lists of weights (in kilograms) of patients from two emergency departments:

Department A	77.5	76.3	75.9	76.9	75.4	75.3	77.0	76.4	77.2	75.9
Department B	56.4	70.3	93.2	45.6	83.9	78.9	88.6	99.6	51.8	95.5

If we want to compare the two groups, it is reasonable to calculate the mean for each group to see if there is any difference between them – we do this by adding each weight and then dividing by the number of subjects:

Department A: Mean = 763.8 ÷ 10 = 76.38 kg
Department B: Mean = 763.8 ÷ 10 = 76.38 kg

So the means are the same, but it seems obvious that to say the two groups are the same is incorrect, and this is highlighted when we list the weights in order of size:

Department A	75.3	75.4	75.9	75.9	76.3	76.4	76.9	77.0	77.2	77.5
Department B	45.6	51.8	56.4	70.3	78.9	83.9	88.6	93.2	98.5	99.6

Clearly, the results from Department A are less spread out than those from Department B. We can give a measure of this by calculating the standard deviation of each sample. Technically, we first calculate what is called the variance and from that we calculate the standard deviation.

CALCULATING VARIANCE

1. Calculate the difference between each data point and the mean:

$$\text{e.g.}\ (x_1 - \bar{x}) + (x_2 - \bar{x}) + (x_3 - \bar{x}) \ldots$$

2. Sort out the problem that if we add those all together, the answer will be zero, as half the results will be positive and half negative.

$$\text{e.g.}\ (x_1 - \bar{x})^2 + (x_2 - \bar{x})^2 + (x_3 - \bar{x})^2 \ldots$$

3. Divide by the number in the sample −1:

$$\left[\sum (x_1 - \bar{x})^2\right] / (n - 1)$$

CALCULATING THE STANDARD DEVIATION

$$\text{Standard deviation} = \sqrt{\text{Variance}} = \sqrt{\frac{\sum (x_1 - \bar{x})^2}{n - 1}}$$

KEY: WHAT DO ALL THESE SYMBOLS MEAN?

The symbols in the equations are mathematical shorthand and are supposed to make things easier, For clarity:

x = any bit of data
x_1 = first bit of data, x_2 = second bit of data, and so on
Σ = 'sum of' (i.e. add everything together)
$\bar{x}$ = mean of all the data
n = total number of pieces of data
$\sqrt{}$ = square root

EXAMPLE

So, let's first calculate the standard deviation of the weights of Department A.

1. Calculate the variance:

$$\frac{\begin{array}{l}(75.3-76.38)^2+(75.4-76.38)^2+(75.9-76.38)^2+(76.3-76.38)^2\\(76.4-76.38)^2+(76.9-76.38)^2+(77.0-76.38)^2\\+(77.2-76.38)^2+(77.5-76.38)^2\end{array}}{(10-1)}$$

Variance = 0.58

2. Calculate the standard deviation:

$$\begin{aligned}\text{Standard deviation} &= \sqrt{\text{Variance}}\\ &= \sqrt{0.58}\\ &= 0.76\,\text{kg}\end{aligned}$$

If we were to perform the same calculation to find the standad deviation of the weights of Department B, we would find it is 19.40 kg. Therefore although the means of the two groups are the same, the standard deviations of the two groups are very different, thus highlighting that there is an important difference between the two groups.

INFERENCES ABOUT THE WHOLE POPULATION FROM SAMPLE DATA

It is important to understand that from a single sample (a set of observations) you can make inferences about the whole population. The population values are fixed. All we are trying to do by taking a sample is to make an estimate of the population.

If we look at the blood pressure drop achieved in a sample of patients given a new antihypertensive, we are able to measure the mean drop in blood pressure and the spread of the results in our sample, but what we are really interested in is what is likely to happen in the population as a whole if we give them the new drug. This is where statistics can become our friend (really!).

More Reasons Why a Normal Distribution Is So Valuable

The first important point to understand is that normally distributed data has one further mathematical quality which we have not yet discussed: we can guarantee that certain proportions of the results will always fall within certain numbers of standard deviations (SDs) either side of the mean (Figure 3.5). Thus, it is always true that:

- 68% of the results will lie within ±1 SD of the mean (i.e. one SD above and one below the mean)

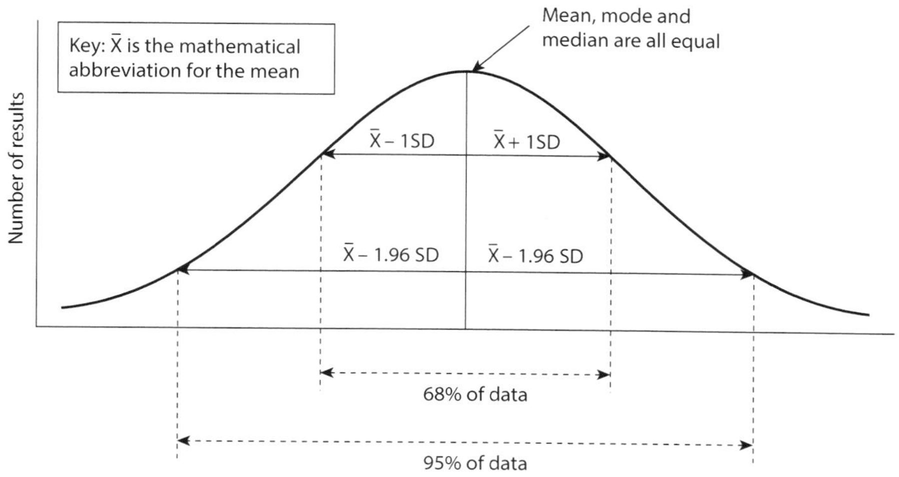

FIGURE 3.5 The proportion of data within various standard deviations of the mean of a normal distribution.

- 95% of the results will lie within ±1.96 SD of the mean (many people will round this up to 2)
- 99% of the results will lie within ±2.5 SD of the mean

A second and equally important feature of normal distributions concerns how we use our sample data set to draw conclusions about the whole population. Let's think about a study looking at the mean height of all the emergency physicians (EPs) in the world. It is impractical to think we could actually measure every EP's height, but we could look to measure the heights of a randomly selected subset of EPs and from this calculate the mean height of that sample. If there are enough people in our sample, it might reflect the whole EP world population, but given random variation it might not. However, if we were to repeat the study so that we had a number of sample groups, we would be able to calculate a mean for each group, and the interesting part is that if we were to plot the means of enough sample groups, these means would themselves fall into a normal distribution. Even more interesting is that this is true even if the data from the whole population does not have a normal distribution (see 'Nerd's Corner').

How Accurate an Estimate of the Population Mean Is Our Sample Mean?

Let's move back to our example about blood pressure reductions – we are interested in not only what happened in our sample group but also what is likely to occur in the whole population. Therefore, we have to ask how accurately does our sample result reflect what we would see if we treated (and measured) the whole population?

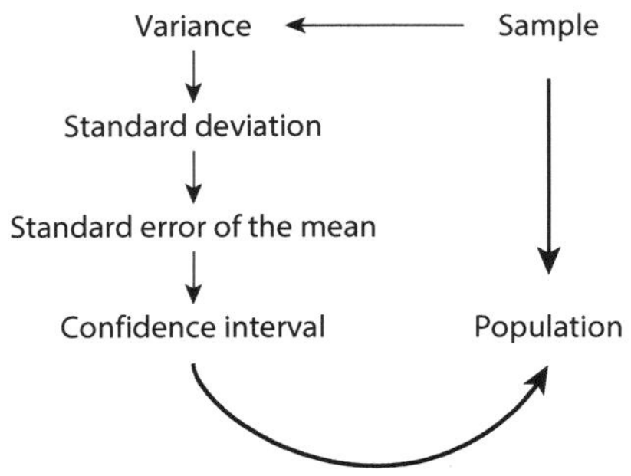

FIGURE 3.6 Making predictions about populations from a single sample.

Intuitively, our sample result is likely to be closer to the population value if:

- The sample is large
- The variation is small

We can also make a reliable estimate of the accuracy of our sample mean compared with the whole population by calculating something called the standard error of the mean (SEM) and using it in a similar way to how we use standard deviation. A fuller explanation of this is given in the following 'Nerd's Corner', but for those who want to keep it simple the following explanation should suffice: We can calculate SEM from the SD of our sample and the number of people within our sample. We can then estimate the accuracy of our sample result compared with the whole population. In a way similar to how 95% of all our sample values fall within 1.96 SD of the mean, we infer that 95% of all the means in all the samples will lie within 1.96 SEM of our sample mean. From this, you can understand the idea of confidence intervals (CIs) – a range which is likely to include the true population mean – and we can calculate them from a single sample.

The flow chart in Figure 3.6 demonstrates a simplification of how we move from the result we obtain from a single sample of patients to draw conclusions about an entire population.

Nerd's Corner

1. If we repeat the study a number of times and the studies are large enough ($N > 30$), we can calculate the means from each of the studies and they will themselves fall into a normal distribution (Figure 3.7).
2. The same rule applies as with any normal distribution: 95% of values will fall within 1.96 SD of the mean. The difference is that when we are moving from a sample mean to estimate a population mean, we do not call it 'standard deviation'; we call it 'standard error of the mean' (Figure 3.8).

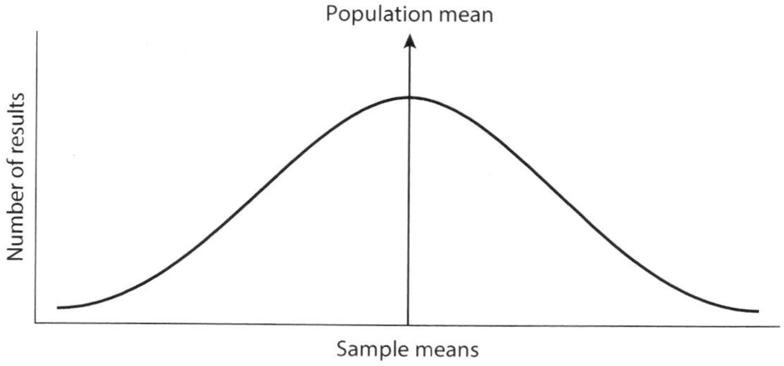

FIGURE 3.7

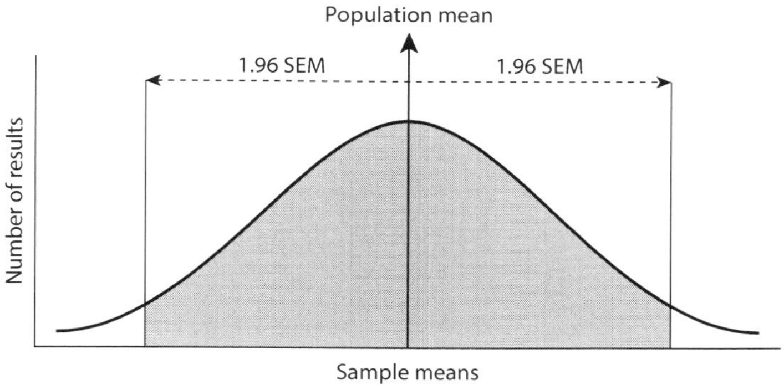

FIGURE 3.8

3. Calculating the standard error of the mean.

$$\text{Standard error of the mean} = \frac{\text{Standard deviation}}{\sqrt{n}}$$

   It is worth noting that if you want to halve the size of your SEM (and hence your CI), you need to quadruple the number of people in your sample.

4. Formal definitions of 95% CIs can often be confusing – we find the following the easiest way to explain them. Imagine taking 100 equally sized samples from a population and calculating means and SEMs for each. Then we can calculate for each sample the 95% CI (sample mean ± 1.96 × SEM). Ninety-five percent of the CIs will contain the true population mean (Figure 3.9).

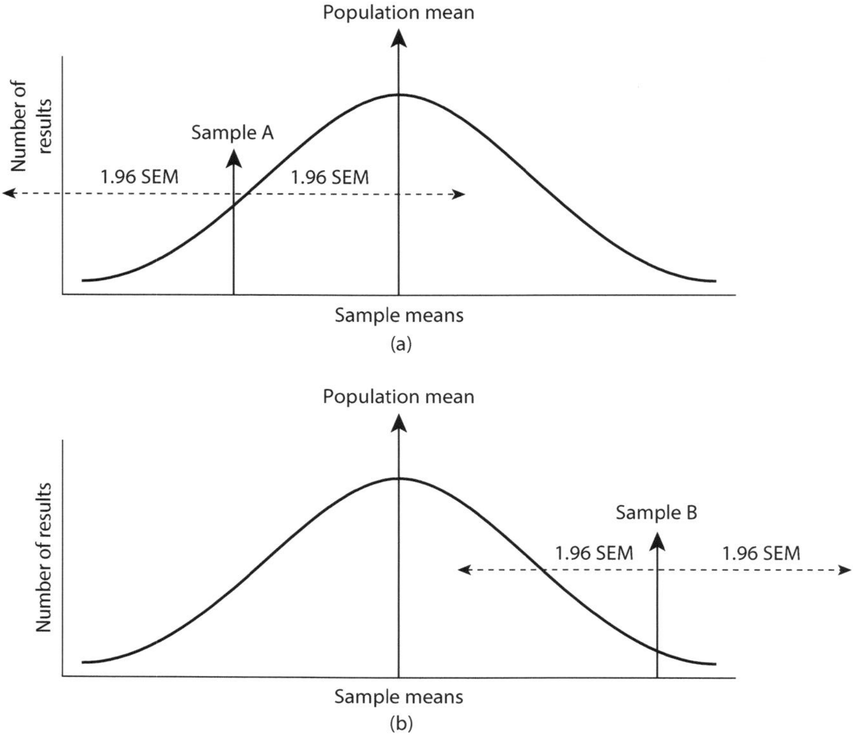

FIGURE 3.9 95% confidence interval = sample mean ± 1.96 SEM. (a) 95% of CIs will contain the population mean, but (b) 5% of CIs will not.

Take-Home Message

From a sample of data we can calculate the mean (a measure of location, or centrality) and the standard deviation (a measure of spread). From this standard deviation we can calculate a standard error of the mean and from this estimate a range which is likely to include the true population mean. This is called the 95% confidence interval for the population mean.

4 The Statistics Used in Papers

Although when you read papers you might be struck by an overabundance of statistical terms, the truth is that what you actually need to know is thankfully a fairly small amount. In this chapter, we cover:

1. Significance
2. Hypothesis testing, p-values and confidence intervals (CIs)
3. Error – or what if the researchers are wrong?
4. Statistical power and how many people are needed in a study
5. Looking out for error in studies
6. Statistical tests

WHAT IS SIGNIFICANCE?

We talk a lot in scientific studies about 'significance', but it is important to realize there are two types of significance: statistical significance and clinical significance. Imagine a study looking at a new antihypertensive that showed a drop in blood pressure of 2 mmHg in the treatment group. We could perform a statistical analysis and might find that the result is *statistically significant*. By this we mean that we think the result demonstrates a difference between the two groups that is unlikely to have occurred by chance. However, it would be reasonable for you to ask whether, in the real world, a drop of 2 mmHg in blood pressure was of any real value, and in doing so you would be questioning the *clinical significance* of the result.

HYPOTHESIS TESTING, P-VALUES AND CONFIDENCE INTERVALS

Hypothesis Testing

When authors embark on a study they will have begun with a research hypothesis. For example, we may have observed that people given aspirin at the time of their acute myocardial infarction (AMI) seem to do better than those who were not, and so we start with a research hypothesis of 'aspirin is better than placebo in AMI'. In superiority trials, we always set up the study so that the default position is we expect that there is no difference between two groups (even if this is not what we actually expect). This is called the *null hypothesis* (H_0). The alternative hypothesis, or study hypothesis (H_1), is the statement that there is a difference between the two groups.

In our example, the null hypothesis is that there is no difference in mortality between patients given aspirin or a placebo for AMI. The study hypothesis is that there is a difference in mortality between patients taking aspirin or a placebo.

We then set about running an experiment and using statistics to help us either reject or not reject the null hypothesis. The slightly awkward 'reject or not reject' is important because even if we reject the null hypothesis, we can say we support the original hypothesis (that aspirin is good for you in AMI). If we do not reject the hypothesis, we are not saying that the null hypothesis is correct; we are just saying that there is not enough evidence to say it is false. This is similar to being found 'not guilty' rather than 'innocent' in a court of law. The answer to whether we reject the null hypothesis can really only be yes or no. This is called *hypothesis testing.*

In hypothesis testing we are asking a yes or no question: Is there a difference, yes or no?

With hypothesis testing, we use statistics to generate a p-value and if it is above or below a predetermined value (by convention 5%, or 0.05), we say that we can either reject or not reject the null hypothesis.

p-Values

We calculate a p-value to enable us to decide if we will reject or not reject the null hypothesis. If we see a difference in mortality rates between our two AMI groups (aspirin and placebo), we need to be aware that while the difference might have occurred because of the treatment, it might also have occurred by chance. In calculating a p-value we are trying to answer the question: How likely are we to have obtained our results if we had sampled from a population where there was no difference between the groups (i.e. if the null hypothesis were true)? The higher the p-value, the more likely that any difference we saw between the groups occurred by chance.

A formal definition of a p-value can be given as:

A p-value is the probability of obtaining a result at least as extreme as the one observed, assuming the null hypothesis is true. The lower the p-value, the less likely the result is if the null hypothesis is true (and the less likely the result is to have occurred by chance).

For many people, that is a bit of a mouthful, and so we prefer:

$p < 0.05$ means that the probability of obtaining the result by chance was less than 1 in 20. By convention, a p-value of less than 0.05 is the accepted threshold for statistical significance and is the level at which the null hypothesis can be rejected.

Example

We want to know if a new painkiller is effective in minor injuries, and we run a study to compare the pain scores in 100 people given the new painkiller versus 100 given just paracetamol. Each patient has a visual analogue pain score on arrival and 1 hour post-analgesia. We can calculate the drop in pain score for each patient, average this out for each group and arrive at a mean pain reduction score for each group: 5 in the treatment group and 2 in the paracetamol group. We can then use a statistical test to calculate a p-value, which in this example comes out as $p = 0.01$.

Because the p-value is less than 0.05, we can say that the result is statistically significant.

Confidence Intervals

Although a simple yes or no answer is sometimes attractive to busy clinicians, in most situations we prefer a bit more information. Many studies are set up so that the information they provide is a measurement. In our example of aspirin in AMI, we might be looking at a mortality rate that could be quoted as a percentage. In that example it is naturally of interest to us what the actual mortality rate in each group was. The result of one sample can only give us an estimation of the result we would get if we were to look at the whole population. However, we can use the results from a single sample, and with statistical testing estimate how accurate our result is in comparison to the whole population.

> A CI provides the reader with a range of plausible values for the true population value. A 95% confidence is the standard size CI used in the medical literature when reporting results. In the same way, a value of less than 0.05 is taken as the threshold of significance when using p-values in hypothesis testing.

Nerd's Corner

Although 95% CIs are commonly thought of as representing the range that has a 95% chance of containing the true (overall population) value, this is sadly not statistically strictly true (sadly, because this is easy to understand). In fact, a 95% CI means that if we were to repeat our experiment ad infinitum and were to construct 95% CIs from each of our sample values, 95% of those intervals would contain the true population value.

It is self-evident and logical that the narrower the CI, the more precise our sample result is in comparison to the overall population result, and thus the more accurate our result.

Confidence intervals can be used in a number of ways:

- Assessing the clinical significance of a result.
    - If the mean drop in blood pressure seen with a new antihypertensive is 10 mmHg, we might feel this is clinically significant. If the 95% CI is 8–12 mmHg, we would agree that even if the true population result was at the lower end (8 mmHg), this would be a clinically significant drop. However, if the 95% CI was 2–18 mmHg, we would probably agree that if the true population result was only 2 mmHg, this would not be clinically significant. Therefore, we must always interpret the mean value alongside the 95% CI to assess clinical significance.
- If we are simply comparing two groups and want to see if there is a real difference between them (i.e. did not occur by chance), we can look to see if the CIs of each group overlap. If they overlap, the result is likely not to be statistically significant.
- If we are looking at a ratio between two groups (e.g. an odds ratio or risk ratio), if the CI crosses 1 (the point of no difference), the result is not statistically significant.

p-Values versus Confidence Intervals

Some studies publish both p-values and CIs, some just one and some just the other, but both p-values and CIs tell us about statistical significance; so is one better than the other? Confidence intervals give us more information, whether the result is statistically significant or not, while allowing us an idea of where the true value might lie (and hence helping us to make a decision about clinical significance). We think CIs are of more use than p-values but in an ideal world, all studies would give both.

Example

In the same analgesia study described earlier, we calculate the mean drop in pain score for each group, but we also calculate the 95% CI for each group. In the treatment group the reduction was 5 with a 95% CI from 4.8 to 5.2 (written as '95% CI 4.8–5.2'), and in the paracetamol group 2 (95% CI 1.8–2.8). As the CIs in each group do not overlap, we can be confident that the difference between the two groups is real, that is, statistically significant.

ERROR – OR WHAT IF THE RESEARCHERS ARE WRONG?

By convention, we say a result is statistically significant if the probability it occurred by chance is less than 5%, and we write this as '$p < 0.05$'. (Ideally the exact value should be given.) It is possible, although unlikely, that a result we take to be statistically significant has in fact occurred by chance. Equally, and for a number of reasons we will later discuss, the results from our study might *not* be statistically significant when in fact there is a difference between the two groups. If any of these happen, we would describe it as an 'error', which we divide into what we call type 1 and type 2 errors (Table 4.1).

Type 1 Error

Making a type 1 error is saying there is a difference between two groups when in fact there is not one. Making this error might lead you to recommend a treatment to patients that is of no benefit to them.

TABLE 4.1
Type 1 and Type 2 Errors

	Alternative Hypothesis Is True (There Is a Difference between the Groups) +ve	Null Hypothesis Is True (There Is No Difference between the Groups) –ve
Experiment shows a significant result, +ve	True positive No error	False positive Type 1 error
Experiment shows no significant result, –ve	False negative Type 2 error	True negative No error

In statistics, we say the probability of making a type 1 error is called alpha (α). We do not actually know the probability of making a type 1 error before we start our experiment, but we can state what we consider to be an acceptable probability of making a type 1 error. This is usually taken to be 5% (or in mathematical terms, 0.05). Alpha is also called the 'threshold for statistical significance'.

It is important we set α before we start our experiment (usually at 0.05) but calculate our p-value once we have our results (and say the result is statistically significant if it is below 0.05). The lower we set α to start with, the lower our p-value needs to be to be statistically significant and the lower the chance our result is a false positive.

Type 2 Error

Making a type 2 error is saying there is no difference between two groups when in fact one is present. This might lead us to withholding a treatment to our patients that in fact would be of benefit to them. Usually, this is due to either the variance in the sample being too great or the sample size being too small.

In statistics, we label the probability of making a type 2 error beta (β). For a fixed sample size, we can consider α and β to be balanced on either end of a set of scales – as we set α (the chance of a false positive result) lower, we make β (the chance of a false negative result) larger. The reason that α is usually set at 0.05 is that conventionally this is taken as a reasonable balancing point. All clinical trials are a balance of the risk of a type 1 error, a type 2 error and sample size.

STATISTICAL POWER AND HOW MANY PEOPLE DO I NEED IN MY STUDY?

Statistical Power

We can describe how likely a study is to detect a difference if one truly exists by subtracting the probability of a type 2 error (a false negative) from 1. We call this 'statistical power' and as a formula we would write it as $1 - \beta$.

By convention the power of a study should be 80–90%; that is, we allow ourselves a 10–20% chance of not demonstrating a difference if one exists.

Determinants of Statistical Power (Probability of Detecting an Effect When It Truly Exists)

1. Alpha – the threshold of significance. Most commonly this is 0.05 and corresponds with accepting a p-value of 0.05 as the cutoff for statistical significance.
2. The variability of the data (measured by the standard deviation).
3. The minimum difference considered to be clinically significant.
4. The sample size.

Sample Size

A major part of designing any study is working out how many people you need to enter into the trial. If we set the statistical power we are aiming for, which by convention is 80–90%, we can calculate the sample size we need by knowing the other aforementioned three determinants. Alpha is usually also set by convention to be 0.05. The variability of the data is a fundamental feature of the data set, and although obviously you cannot know the variability of your data before you start, you can use previous studies or pilot studies to get a good estimation of what it is likely to be. The minimum clinically significant difference (or minimum clinically important difference [MCID]) should be stated before starting a study and ideally should be taken from an independent source such as another research study. It is important that the MCID is a clinical threshold and is therefore determined by the clinician setting up the study and should be explicitly stated.

Example

In our study looking at the effect of our new painkiller, we need to know how many people we are required to recruit *before* we start the study. We start by asking: What chance of a type 2 error am I willing to accept? Let's say 10% (by convention we would usually accept somewhere between 10% and 20%). That means we are aiming for a power of 90% ($1 - \beta = 1 - 0.1 = 0.9$ [90%]). We then set our type 1 error risk, most commonly set at 5% (i.e. $\alpha = 0.05$; if we find a p-value less than 0.05, we will say the result is statistically significant). Additionally, we decide (perhaps from other studies) what is considered to be the minimum reduction in pain score that is clinically significant; let's say a drop of 1.0 on the visual analogue scale we are using. We may also have obtained an estimation of data variability from previous studies.

Finally, we perform a *power calculation* to determine how many people we need to enrol into our study. Exactly how the power calculation is performed is thankfully beyond the scope of this book, but you should understand that the smaller the sample size, the lower your power will be and the higher the chance of a type 2 error (false negative).

Good-quality studies should describe their sample size/power calculation together with all parameters and constants so an independent reviewer can replicate the results.

LOOKING OUT FOR ERRORS IN STUDIES

Spotting Type 1 Errors

We have described that the chance of a type 1 error (a false positive) corresponds to the p-value level we set for accepting statistical significance. Basing your practice on a positive study result that is in fact a false positive (type 1 error) may result in you giving a treatment to a patient which is of no benefit and may even cause harm. Often, type 1 errors occur due to a flaw with the study, either bias or poor methodology.

If we set α at 0.05, we are saying that we are willing to accept a 5% chance of a false positive and that if the p-value we calculate is under 0.05, we will accept that the result is statistically significant. It is really important to note that this is only true if we are talking about looking at one single result. The more results we look at within one trial, and hence the more p-values we calculate, the greater the chance that one of them will be statistically significant purely by chance. That is, the more statistical tests you perform on one sample, the more likely you are to get a statistically significant result; or the wider the net you cast on the data, the bigger chance you get of catching a significant result; or if you overanalyze your data set, you increase your chance of getting a false positive result.

Example

Consider running our analgesia study again. Let's keep α at 0.05 and hence the p-value we will call statistically significant at $p < 0.05$, but this time instead of only quoting a result for reduction in pain, we will also give results for the following: total number of doses taken, days off work, days until pain-free, days requiring analgesia, time spent in the ED, re-attendance rates at the ED, attendance rates at the GP, length of time needing a splint and overall satisfaction.

When we had only one result, the probability that we might find a statistically significant result by chance was 5%, but now because we have 10 results, the probability that one of them will be statistically significant by chance alone jumps to 40%.

Nerd's Corner

Probability of at least one false positive = 1 − (Probability of no false positives in all 10 tests)
Probability of a false positives for each test = 0.05
Probability of not having a false positive 1 − 0.05 = 0.95

Therefore probability of no false positives in 10 tests = $1 - (0.95)^{10} = 1 - 0.6 = 40\%$

(If multiple tests are done on a single data set, each result is not necessarily independent of the others, and hence the calculation is a little more complicated than above, but the general rule holds true.)

Looking for multiple results from one set of data has been termed *data dredging* and is surprisingly common. It is often seen in observational studies and database studies and may reflect a poorly planned study. Equally, the risk of a type 1 error should be particularly watched for when authors report positive results from a subgroup analysis of a study. It is possible to power your study to allow for subgroup analyses and equally statistical correction can be done (e.g. the Bonferroni correction) to account for doing a number of tests on a data set. If neither of these has been done, you should be very wary of authors looking for a positive subgroup result from a trial that overall did not show a statistically significant difference.

Questions to Ask to Avoid Missing a Type 1 Error

- Are there multiple hypothesis tests (are the authors asking more than one question)?
- Is this a subgroup analysis? (In ISIS-2, a famous cardiology study, subdividing patients by astrological sign suggested aspirin had a slightly adverse effect on mortality in Gemini patients but was beneficial in all other star signs.)
- Do the authors report and discuss the results they said they were going to look for in the design of the study?
- Does the result make sense in the context of other known results?

Spotting Type 2 Errors

Type 2 errors are what occur when we fail to find a statistically significant result when a real difference was actually present. When a type 2 error occurs, it is usually because the sample size was too small.

In studies that reported a non-statistically significant result it is easy to dismiss the study and conclude that the intervention that was studied is of no value. This risks missing the fact that valuable information can be gained from assessing whether a type 2 error may have caused a negative result and whether in fact you should still keep an open mind about the treatment or diagnostic test the authors looked at.

Questions to Ask to Avoid Missing a Type 2 Error

- How wide are the CIs? (If they are very wide, this suggests the sample size was too small and hence there might be a type 2 error.)
- Do the CIs encompass a potentially clinically important difference?
- Did the authors perform a power calculation and were all the variables included appropriately calculated/estimated?
- Was the minimum clinically important difference the authors set actually too big?

TYPES OF STATISTICAL TESTS

Statistical tests are used mainly to make inferences about a population from which the sample was taken. We can use statistics to:

- Look at the differences between samples
- Look for equivalence and non-inferiority
- Look for correlations between groups

To decide which statistical test is the most appropriate you need the following information:

- How many groups do you need to compare?
- What type of data do you have?

- What type of distribution does the data produce?
- Do you need to adjust for confounders?

Once you have this information you can use Figure 4.1 to figure out the appropriate test. These tests can then be used to calculate a p-value. It is important to understand what a p-value is and where it is of use, but you do not need to know how you calculate that value. Knowledge of the statistical test and when you should use each type is useful for when reading papers.

Statistical methods can be used to assess relationships. We call this correlation and regression. Correlation assesses the strength of the relationship between two variables. The correlation coefficient is the measurement of this relationship although it does not measure causation. Types of correlation include Pearson's, Spearman's rank and Kendall's.

R-Value	Degree of Correlation
–1	(Perfect) negative correlation
0	No correlation
1	Perfect correlation

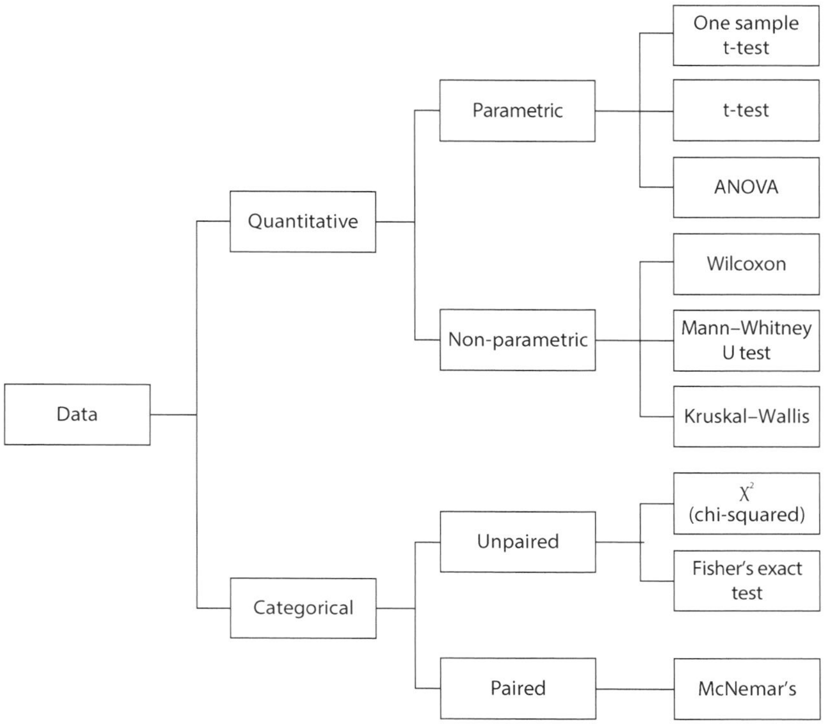

FIGURE 4.1 Statistical tests depending on data type.

When you have a relationship between two things, you can plot this relationship on a graph. Regression determines the nature of the relationship between the two variables. It is possible that multiple factors can affect the relationship and in that case, multiple regression analysis is used.

Take-Home Message

1. The difference between p-values and CIs and the fact that we think CIs are more valuable.

p-Value	Confidence Interval
Needs a statement at the start of the study about what the authors think is *clinically significant*	Allows the reader to interpret the size of the result and helps determine whether it is *clinically significant*
Gives a yes or no answer to whether the result is significant	Gives a plausible range for the true population value

2. Type 1 error = False positive rate; Type 2 error = False negative rate.
3. The necessary sample size of a study is calculated from: the power of the study (set before you start the study and usually 80–90%), the predicted variability of the data and the minimum difference that is deemed clinically significant. In a good-quality scientific paper the power calculation should be described by the authors with sufficient details so that the reader can replicate it.

5 Basic Probability

It may seem strange to have a chapter on A-level mathematics in a medical textbook, but it is important to understand probability and odds when reading the results section of a paper. We understand that for some people this part of critical appraisal can be challenging and off-putting, but please stick with it. We have kept it as brief as possible and with the clinical significance highlighted.

PROBABILITY

Unless you like betting on horses or dogs, probabilities are much more intuitive than odds.

- Probability is the likelihood of any event happening as a proportion of the total number of possibilities. Or put more simply:

  Probability = Number of desired events ÷ Total possible number of events

- The probability of something which is certain to happen is 1.
- The probability of an impossible event is 0.
- Probability can easily be turned into a percentage by multiplying by 100; therefore a probability of 1 can also be described as a probability of 100%.
- Probability is a way of expressing risk or chance.

Let's give some simple examples.

Example 1: A Coin

- When I toss a coin, there are two possibilities: heads or tails.
- The probability of a head is 1 ÷ 2, which equals 0.5, or 50%.

Example 2: A Dice

- When I roll a dice, there are six potential outcomes: 1, 2, 3, 4, 5 or 6.
- I have a one in six chance of getting a 6: 1 ÷ 6 = 0.167, or 16.7%.

Risk versus Probability

Risk is calculated in the same way as probability, and to all intents and purposes the definition of risk is identical. Therefore, when we look at therapeutic papers, we can work out the risk in the control group and the experimental group.

Experimental event rate (EER) is just another way of saying risk in the experimental group, that is, the number of patients who had the experimental treatment and died (if that is the outcome of interest we are looking at) divided by the total number who had the experimental treatment.

Likewise, control event rate (CER) is just another way of saying risk in the control group, that is, the number of patients who had the standard treatment and died divided by the total number who had the standard treatment.

One way of assessing the value of the experimental treatment is to compare the two ratios by dividing the EER by the CER; we call this relative risk:

$$\text{Relative Risk} = \frac{\text{Experimental event rate}}{\text{Control evevt rate}}$$

All the other calculations required in the results section of therapeutic papers (e.g. absolute risk reduction or number needed to treat) are based on these simple calculations. This is discussed in greater detail in Chapter 8 on therapeutic papers.

Nerd's Corner: A Bit More about Probabilities

Probabilities can be used in three ways:

1. The probability of something not happening is 1 minus the probability that it will happen:
   i.e. the probability of anything but a 6 when I roll a dice is 1 – 1/6

   = 5/6 = 0.83 = 83%

2. The probability of either one event or another event happening is the probability of each event happening added to each other:
   i.e. the probability of a 6 or a 5 is the probability of a 5 plus the probability of a 6

   = 1/6 + 1/6 = 1/3 = 0.33 = 33%

3. The probability of an event happening and then another independent event happening = probability of each event happening multiplied together:
   i.e. the probability of a 6 and then another 6 is 1/6 times 1/6

   = 1/36 = 0.028 = 2.8%

ODDS

So, if probabilities are so easy to understand, why do we also use odds?

Before looking at why we use odds, let's get an understanding of them first. They are a lot less intuitive than probabilities (and perhaps this is why they are used by bookmakers).

Odds are calculated as:

Odds = desired events ÷ undesired events

- The odds of something certain to happen are infinity.
- The odds of an impossible event are 0.

Let's give some simple examples.

Example 1: A Coin

- When I toss a coin, there are two possibilities: heads or tails.
- The odds of a head are 1:1.

Example 2: A Dice

- When I throw a dice, there are six potential outcomes: 1, 2, 3, 4, 5 or 6.
- The odds of a 6 are 1:5.

(See 'Nerd's Corner: Converting Probabilities to Odds and Vice Versa' later in this chapter.)

Odds in Therapeutic Trials

Odds can be used to look at outcomes in therapeutic trials. For example, the odds in the treatment group of a trial are calculated by the number of patients who received the new intervention and died (if that was the outcome of interest) divided by the number who received the new intervention and did not die.

Similarly, the odds in the control group of a trial are calculated by the number of patients who received the control treatment (standard treatment) and died divided by the number who received the control treatment (standard treatment) and did not die.

In exactly the same way as risk, we can compare the odds in the two groups by calculating a ratio.

Odds ratio = Odds in treated group ÷ Odds in control group

ODDS VERSUS PROBABILITY (RISK)

We asked earlier why we need to worry about odds when probabilities seem easier to understand. We will start answering that by showing how odds and probabilities compare in a couple of examples.

Trial A

	Dead	Alive
New treatment	100	900
Control treatment	500	500

EER = 100/1000 = 0.1	Experimental odds = 100/900 = 0.11
CER = 500/1000 = 0.5	Control odds = 500/500 = 1
RR = 0.1/0.5 = 0.2	Odds ratio = 0.11/1 = 0.11

Trial B

	Dead	Alive
New treatment	1	999
Control treatment	5	995

EER = 1/1000 = 0.001	Experimental odds = 1/999 = 0.001001
CER = 5/1000 = 0.005	Control odds = 5/995 = 0.005025
RR = 0.001/0.005 = 0.2	Odds ratio = 0.001001/0.005025 = 0.199

It can be seen that when events are rare, risk and odds are similar. But as the prevalence increases, then the odds ratios and risk ratios become very different. It is easy to see that you might choose one over the other to present a particular slant to the results from your trial – this is shown in the example in the following 'Nerd's Corner'.

Nerd's Corner: Odds Ratios Appearing to Exaggerate Claims

Consider the following (fictional) data on nursing exam pass rates:

	Fail	Pass	Total
Male	33	14	47
Female	16	72	88
Total	49	86	135

It is obvious that a female candidate was more likely to pass than a male candidate, but the question is, *how much more likely?* You could work out either the relative risk or the odds ratio to answer this question.

The odds ratio compares the relative odds of passing in each group. The odds of men passing were 14/33 = 0.42, but for women 72/16 = 4.5. The odds ratio is therefore calculated to be 10.7 (4.5/0.42); that is, there is a more than 10-fold greater odds of passing for females than for males.

The relative risk (also called the risk ratio) compares the probability (risk) of passing in each group rather than the odds. For males, the probability of passing is 30% (14/47 = 0.3), while for females, the probability (risk) is 82% (72/88 = 0.82). The relative risk of passing is 2.7 (0.82/0.3); that is, there is a 2.7 greater probability of passing for females than for males.

We can see there is a massive difference between the odds ratio and the relative risk and this can confuse people. Both measurements show that men were more likely to fail, but the odds ratio implies that men are much worse off than the relative risk. Which number is a fairer comparison? We would argue that as the risk ratio is the simplest to understand, it should usually be used unless there is a specific reason to use the odds ratio. As we have demonstrated, be aware that the odds ratio might sometimes be used to inflate the difference.

Given that risk (probability) is intuitively more easily understood, we would suggest these should be given most often in the results of a study. So why do we use (and need to understand) both? Odds essentially have 'superior mathematical properties', which make them very useful.

Odds Having Superior Mathematical Properties

There are three main areas where odds are superior to risk (probability), but the key one is in diagnostic papers and calculating post-test probabilities. The other two areas where odds are better are shown in the 'Nerd's Corner' below.

Nerd's Corner: Other Uses of Odds

ODDS IN META-ANALYSIS

Relative risk depends on the prevalence of the disease being studied, but odds ratios do not. So if you are comparing multiple trials with differing prevalence in each trial, then combining relative risks is not mathematically sound, but combining odds ratios is.

ODDS IN CASE CONTROL STUDIES

In case control studies, the researchers define how many patients there are with and without the disease; that is, they define their own prevalence. It therefore is not appropriate to use a calculation (risk ratio or relative risk) that is influenced by prevalence.

Calculating Post-Test Probabilities Using Odds

The rest of this chapter covers the mathematics behind how we use investigations to make diagnoses in medicine: the 'Bayesian theory of medicine' in practice. This is an important concept to grasp in preparation for Chapter 9 on diagnostic papers.

You may not know exactly what Bayesian theory means – but you do it every day. When we see a patient, we make an estimate of how likely they are to have a specific condition. We do this using our clinical 'gestalt' (or in other words, the combination of our clinical skills and experience, the patient's demographics, and their history and examination combined with the population prevalence). This is the pre-test probability of a patient having the condition.

We may then do a test to help us decide if the patient has the condition in question. Unfortunately, tests are not perfect and a yes or no test result will invariably not give us a 100% definitive answer. What the test actually does is help us decide the probability of the patient having the condition: the post-test probability.

Each test has a likelihood ratio attached to it, that is, how much more likely a positive test is to be found in a person with the disease than in a patient without the disease. The post-test probability is the pre-test probability combined with the likelihood ratio.

There are likelihood ratios for positive tests (which range from 1 upwards – the higher it is, the better the test) and there are likelihood ratios for negative test results (which range from 0 to 1 – with the closer to zero, the better the test).

We may not realize it, but we do estimations of this calculation every single time we see a patient. While we are taking our history, we are making an estimate of the patient's pre-test probability. When we examine them we refine our probability. When we get a test result back, we use our knowledge of that test – our personal estimate of the likelihood ratio – to see how likely they are to have the condition. For example, in someone who we are concerned may have a pulmonary embolism, the patient's management will depend more often than not on the computed tomography pulmonary angiogram (CTPA) and not necessarily on the D-dimer. This is because the likelihood ratio of a CTPA is greater than that of a D-dimer for the diagnosis of a pulmonary embolism.

If we are trying to put actual numbers onto these post-test probabilities, as opposed to just estimates, then we must use odds and not probabilities. We can only calculate post-test probabilities by going via odds.

To get from pre-test probability to post-test probability, we go through a number of steps:

1. Convert pre-test probability to pre-test odds.
2. Multiply pre-test odds by the likelihood ratio to calculate post-test odds.
3. Convert post-test odds to post-test probability.

This all seems like a bit of a faff, but let's look at why we need to do it. Remember, probabilities can only go from 0 to 1, but odds go from 0 to infinity. If we multiply the (positive) likelihood ratio with a probability, we may often get a number greater than 1, which in terms of probabilities makes no sense at all.

Let's look at an example:

- We are looking after a trauma patient.
- We suspect he has an 80% chance of a pneumothorax.
- We perform an ultrasound, which has a likelihood ratio of 9; that is, we are nine times more likely to diagnose a pneumothorax by ultrasound in someone who has one as opposed to someone who does not. (Remember, each operator will have a different likelihood ratio for subjective tests such as ultrasound, based on their skills and competencies.)
- Once you have the ultrasound result, now what is the chance of having a pneumothorax?
- Using probabilities:
  - Post-test probability = Pre-test probability combined with the likelihood ratio
  - Pre-test probability: 80%, mathematically written as 0.8
  - Likelihood ratio = 9
- Post-test probability would be $0.8 \times 9 = 7.2$
- In probability terms this makes no sense: remember that a probability of 1.0 (100%) means something is absolutely certain to happen. In this example the result works out as 7.2, or 720%, and clearly this does not make sense.
- Using odds:
  - (Pre-test) odds = 80:20 = 4:1 (based on probability of 80%)

- Likelihood ratio = 9
- Post-test odds = Pre-test odds × Likelihood ratio = 4:1 × 9 = 36:1

- Odds of 36:1 clearly makes sense (suggesting a very high chance of having a pneumothorax given a positive ultrasound).

Converting Post-Test Odds to Probabilities

We can see that if we are doing tests, we need to use odds. But the 36:1 post-test odds of having a pneumothorax are not intuitive. We need to convert it to a probability (which can be expressed as a percentage). There are two ways of doing this.

The first is by using mathematics. In the following 'Nerd's Corner', we show how you go from probability to odds and back again. But you must remember that it is not necessary to know these formulae, and they are there just for those who have an excessive interest in odds and probabilities.

Nerd's Corner: Converting Probabilities to Odds and Vice Versa

CONVERTING PROBABILITY TO ODDS

$$\text{Odds} = \text{Probability} \div (1 - \text{Probability})$$

Let's take the example of the coin:

- The probability of a head is 0.5 and the odds = 0.5/(1 – 0.5) = 0.5/0.5 = 1, which is written as 1:1.

Let's take the example of a dice:

- The probability of a 6 is 0.1667.
- The odds = 0.167/(1 – 0.167) = 0.167/0.83 = 1/5, which is written as 1:5.

Let's take the example of the pneumothorax pre-test probability:

- The pre-test probability of a pneumothorax is 0.8. The pre-test odds of a pneumothorax are thus 0.8:0.2 = 4:1.

CONVERTING ODDS TO PROBABILITY

$$\text{Probability} = \text{Odds} \div (\text{Odds} + 1)$$

Let's take the example of the coin:

- The odds of a head are 1:1 and the probability = 1/(1 + 1) = 0.5 (50%).

Let's take the example of a dice:

- The odds of a 6 are 1:5. The probability = 1/(5 + 1) = 0.167 (16.7%).

Let's take the example of the pneumothorax post-test odds:

- The odds are 36:1. The probability is thus 36/(36 + 1) = 0.973 (97.3%).

Converting Post-Test Odds to Probability the Easy Way (by Just Knowing the Pre-Test Probability and Likelihood Ratio)

The second way of doing this – with much less effort – uses a nomogram. It very accurately calculates the post-test probability using the pre-test probability and the likelihood ratio by drawing one straight line. All the complicated sums of converting probability to odds, multiplying by likelihood ratio and then converting post-test odds to post-test probability have already been done for us. All we need to do is plot the pre-test probability and the likelihood ratio and then draw the line (Figure 5.1).

We draw a line from a point on the left-hand line, from where our clinical gestalt tells us the pre-test probability lies, through the likelihood ratio for the test, and extend it on to the post-test probability. Where it cuts this line is the patient's post-test probability.

We have to remember that the post-test probability is really an estimate, based on a best guess pre-test probability and the likelihood ratio, which if it is a subjective test such as an ultrasound, is user dependent. The beauty of the nomogram is that the same one can be used for all diseases and all tests.

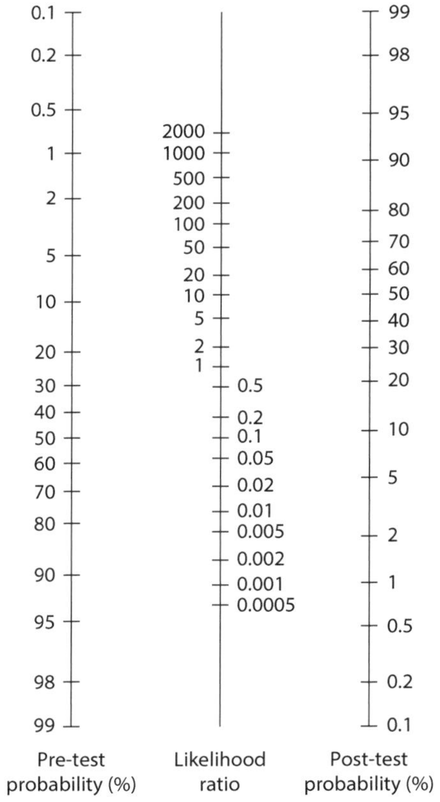

FIGURE 5.1 The nomogram for converting pre-test probabilities and likelihood ratios to post-test probabilities.

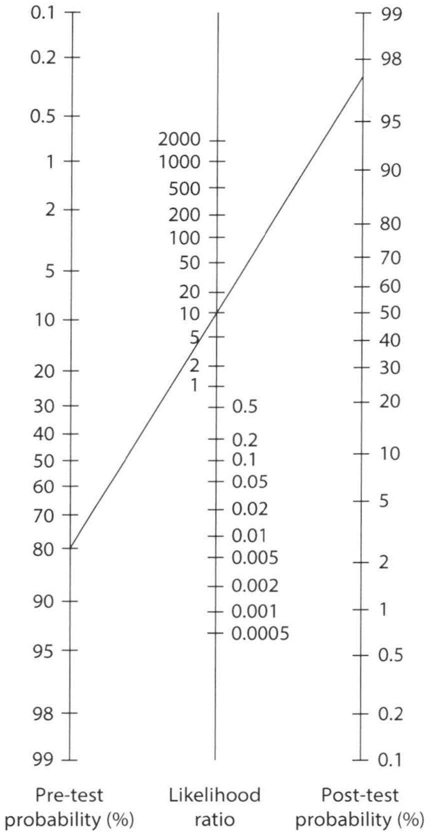

FIGURE 5.2 The nomogram for converting pre-test probabilities to post-test probabilities for pneumothorax. Pre-test probability = 0.8; likelihood ratio = 9. Post-test probability = 0.973 (97.3%), which is the same as the calculated post-test probability shown in 'Nerd's Corner'.

Let's look at how we would use the nomogram for the pneumothorax example we used previously. As long as the line and intercepts are drawn accurately, then the post-test probability is accurate (Figure 5.2).

Take-Home Message

1. Odds and probability are two ways of expressing the chance of something happening, but they are not interchangeable. Probabilities are easier to understand than odds and in appropriate situations should be used in preference to odds.
2. Bayesian theory is the process of using the likelihood ratio of a test to move from pre-test probability to post-test probability.

Section 3

Appraising Different Types of Papers

6 Observational Studies

Let's now move on and discuss critically appraising observational studies. As we described in Chapter 1, observational studies are usually considered a lower grade of evidence than randomized interventional trials, and this may be the reason that often less time is given to how to appraise observational trials. Nevertheless, observational trials make up a significant proportion of the literature and a number of highly important advances have been made on the back of observational data – an often-quoted example being the British Doctors Study in the 1950s, which demonstrated the association between smoking and lung cancer. As such, we believe a good understanding of how to appraise them is very important.

INTERNAL VERSUS EXTERNAL VALIDITY

As with all studies, and as we covered previously, we recommend you consider the appraisal of any study on the basis of internal and external validity. For most of this chapter we will focus on the internal validity of the various observational studies, but consideration of external validity is no less important.

When thinking about external validity, ask whether the researchers have asked a question that is relevant to your area of practice, covering an intervention, risk factor or outcome that is of interest to you and in a population that would mean that the result would be generalizable to the sorts of patients you routinely encounter. For example, if the study looks only at patients aged 18–50, it will be difficult to generalize this result to an elderly care clinic.

START AT THE BEGINNING: IS THIS AN OBSERVATIONAL TRIAL?

Before you decide on how to appraise any study, first decide what sort of study it is. Figure 6.1 was shown previously in Chapter 1, but when critically appraising observational studies, the first (and sometimes not very easy) step is to recognize that it is an observational rather than an interventional study.

From Chapter 1 and Figure 6.1, we know that in observational studies the researchers do not 'do' anything to the patients or subjects. This does not mean that the patients are not receiving new drugs, operations or tests, but it does mean that the decision about what the patients receive is not made by the researchers; the patients are treated or behave in whatever way they would have done regardless of whether they had been in a study. The researchers merely observe and record what happened at the time and what happens subsequently.

For the rest of this chapter, we are going to break things down, looking at the design, methodology, results and conclusion of observational trials.

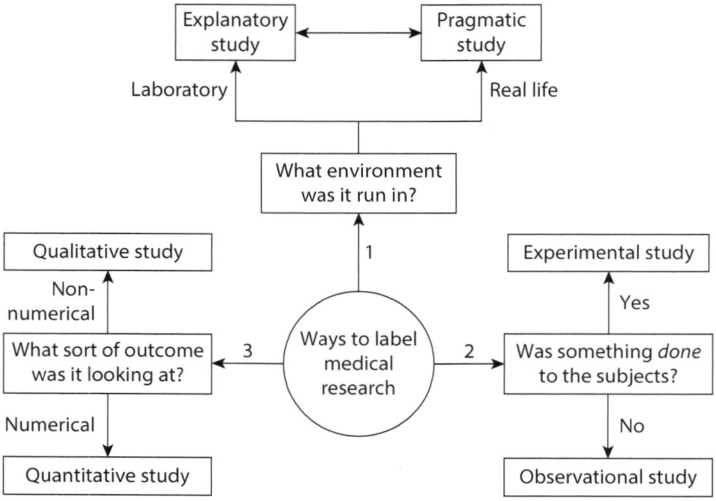

FIGURE 6.1 Different ways to label a trial – three questions to ask.

DESIGN

Once you have worked out that you are dealing with an observational trial, the next thing to look at is the design of the study. This will incorporate what question the researchers were trying to answer and what sort of observational trial they have performed. As ever, a healthy degree of scepticism about why they chose that design of trial is often helpful.

What Question Are the Researchers Asking?

Begin by asking what question the researchers are trying to answer. Can you work this out easily from the title or introduction section of the paper? Many observational trials can be done on data that has already been collected for another reason. However, re-analyzing it simply for the sake of re-analyzing it is not good practice and may well produce falsely positive results (see the section on spotting type 1 errors in Chapter 4).

Where the question that the researchers are asking is either unclear or poorly defined (or even worse, appears to have been structured to fit the data set available), ask yourself whether it is the question that is driving the trial or the availability of the data. Where trials are data driven, be suspicious of the chance of false positive results (type 1 errors).

Is the Trial Design the Right One for the Question That Is Being Asked?

In Chapter 1 we have already made brief mention of the four main types of observational trial: case control, cohort and cross-sectional and ecological trials. Each has its own merits and limitations, and when designing a trial, researchers should use a type of trial that fits the question.

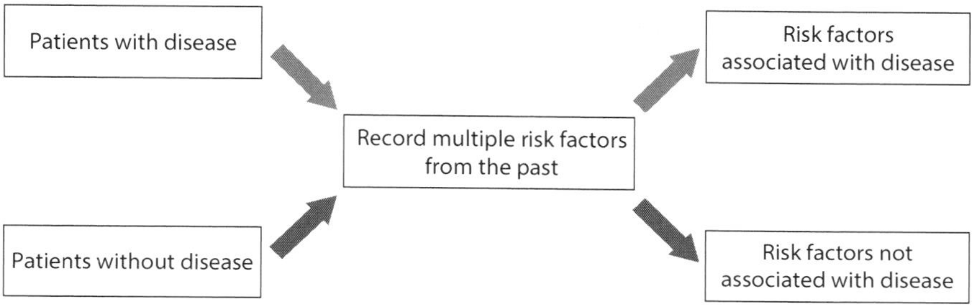

FIGURE 6.2 How case control studies are formulated.

Case Control Studies

What Are They?

In case control studies, the researchers look at a set of patients with a certain disease and ask the question about what risk factors or exposures *might* have caused it. In order to make some suggestions, they match their patients with the disease to patients who do not have the disease and try to find out what each group has been exposed to and the differences between them.

An example would be looking at patients who have developed a particular form of leukaemia. We could match them to a group of people who do not have leukaemia and then research into their past looking at the different things they have been exposed to and whether we can see any obvious differences that might be related to the development of leukaemia. This is shown in Figure 6.2.

In What Situations Are They Good?

Case control studies are good when you are dealing with patients who have a rare disease. They allow you to find and then group together a large enough group of people with their rare disease to allow you a better chance of drawing some conclusions about what similar characteristics and exposures they share, and the ones that are different to patients who do not have the disease.

Why Might They Not Be So Good?

While good at looking at rare diseases, the opposite is true of rare risk factors or exposures. If the risk factor that causes the disease is very rare, you will need to enrol a large number of people to highlight that the risk factor is important. The intrinsically retrospective nature of case control studies is also a significant issue, which we will discuss in the results section of this chapter.

Cohort Studies

What Are They?

In some respects cohort studies can be thought of as the opposite of case control studies. Patients who have been given or exposed to the treatment or risk factor of interest are followed in time to see what happens to them. They are compared to a group (or 'cohort') of patients who were not given or exposed to the

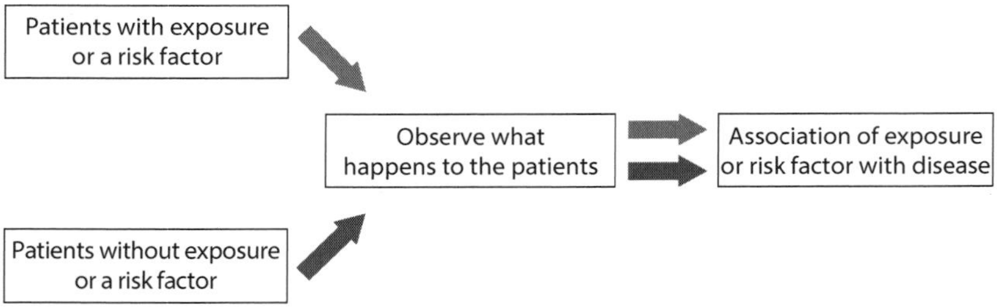

FIGURE 6.3 How cohort studies are formulated.

same treatment or risk factor, and hence the outcomes of the two groups (whether mortality, length of hospital stay or any number of other outcomes) can be compared. See Figure 6.3.

It is also worth highlighting that to some extent this is similar to the interventional 'controlled' trial we discuss in Chapters 1 and 8. However, the important difference to appreciate is that in cohort studies, whether the subjects get or do not get the treatment or risk factor is not up to the researchers; it is merely a feature of the variations in practice or real life that routinely occur.

Cohort studies should ideally be designed around a specific question and run prospectively. However, if a data set already existed (consider a trauma registry with a record of every trauma call a hospital receives and a lot of pre-designated information records on each patient), it would be perfectly possible and reasonable to look retrospectively at a cohort of people from that data set with and without an exposure and what happened to them. We would call that a retrospective cohort study.

We mentioned earlier the British Doctors Study that began in 1956 and ran until 2001. In this study the researchers looked at a group of doctors who smoked and compared them over 4½ decades with doctors who did not. The study was a major step in highlighting the link between smoking and lung cancer and had a major effect on public health policy. Importantly, they did not intervene in the doctors' choice about smoking and certainly did not tell them to smoke or not smoke – that was left up to the doctors. Therefore, the researchers were observing rather than intervening, making this an observational rather than interventional trial.

In What Situations Are They Good?

Cohort studies are particularly valuable when you know the treatment or risk factor you are interested in but want to know about a lot of different outcomes. Remember, the general rules of critical appraisal always apply. Particularly, looking at a lot of outcomes increases the risk that one of them will prove to be statistically significant by chance. The researchers must state all outcomes they are looking at prior to analyzing the data, so to not 'data dredge'. Having too many outcomes being analyzed increases the risk of type 1 errors, as explained in Chapter 4.

Why Might They Not Be So Good?

As we have mentioned, we might consider cohort studies to be the opposite of case control studies, and this is true of the reasons they might not be so good. If we are looking at very rare outcomes, a cohort study will have to include a very large number of patients potentially over a much longer time frame, meaning greater expense. Greater expense is a major restriction on the completion of high-quality research.

We have mentioned earlier and in Chapter 4 the risks of looking at multiple outcomes from one data set, and these should always be borne in mind when looking at cohort studies that look at a number of different outcomes. With retrospective cohort studies, you should consider how many times the data set has been used to look at different questions, and hence make an assessment of the risks of false positive results (type 1 errors).

Cross-Sectional Studies

What Are They?

In cross-sectional studies the researchers look at either exposure or disease, or both, at a single time point (or over a short time period). Information can be gathered from patients via questionnaires or interviews, which allows the possibility of collecting data about a number of exposures, potentially confounding factors and diseases. Therefore, the information for cross-sectional studies is collected from individual subjects. They are most commonly used to demonstrate prevalence (prevalence is the number of people with the disease or risk factor divided by the number of the population studied). See Figure 6.4.

In What Situations Are They Good?

As we say above, cross-sectional studies are good for looking at prevalence, of either a disease or a risk factor, or both. They are relatively cheap and easy to run and are often described as a 'snapshot' of a population. They allow us to build a theory that if there is a high prevalence of an exposure and a high prevalence of a disease, those two things are possibly correlated.

Why Might They Not Be So Good?

Importantly, cross-sectional studies cannot do more to suggest causation as they do not allow the researchers to look at the temporal relationship between risk factor and disease development. Hence, when considering the link between exposure to a risk and the development of a disease, they can only be used to generate a hypothesis to run further studies. Equally, cross-sectional studies do not allow you to calculate

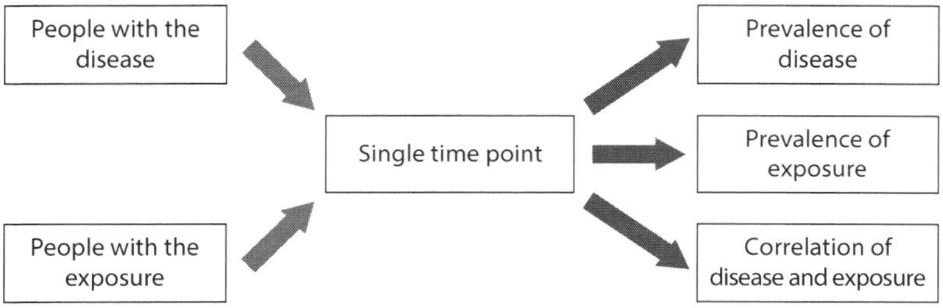

FIGURE 6.4 How cross-sectional studies are formulated.

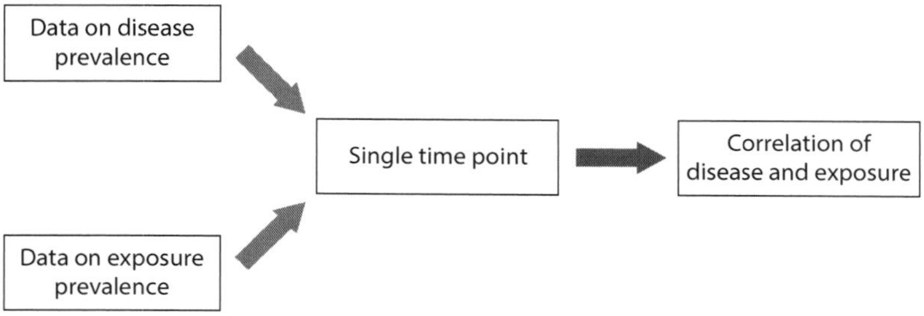

FIGURE 6.5 How ecological studies are formulated.

incidence (the number of new cases that occur in a given time frame, usually a year), as they are designed to look only at one time point (or a very short time period).

Ecological Studies

What Are They?

Ecological studies can be thought of as the most basic sort of observational study, and perhaps the easiest way to describe them is as simplistic cross-sectional studies. Again, the researchers look at the rates of diseases and exposures in a population, but in these studies they do not collect information from individuals and instead use already known or collected population data. Often the data come from published statistics on populations, such as mortality rates or rates of people smoking. By having the data on different populations, it is possible to compare disease and exposure rates between populations, be they different geographical, social or temporal populations. See Figure 6.5.

In What Situations Are They Good?

As we have said, these are considered very basic studies, and they are cheap and easy to run. They are good for generating hypotheses for testing with more complex studies about potential links between an exposure and a disease.

Why Might They Not Be So Good?

Like cross-sectional studies, there is no element of demonstrating temporal flow between exposure to a risk factor and development of a disease, and hence causation cannot be shown by an ecological study. Because these studies are usually done on rates of disease or exposure that are already known, the original data may not be available, meaning the number of people originally studied may not be clear. Equally, unlike with cross-sectional studies, it is unlikely that information on confounders will be available, further reducing the quality of the result.

METHODOLOGY

Now you have decided that this is an observational trial and that the researchers have used the right sort of trial to answer their question, the next thing to do is to look at the methodology of the trial. As always, the things to look out for will depend on the type of trial you are looking at, but common to all trials is to make sure you are happy with the way the researchers have selected the participants in their trial. Equally, all trials should report a rationale behind how many patients they included (as you would do in a power calculation in an interventional trial). By their very nature, no observational trial is randomized, but the rationale and process for how participants were selected should be transparent and fair; if not, the trial is likely to suffer from bias.

Case Control Studies

Who Did They Include and Who Agreed to Take Part?

The first and perhaps the most important question to ask is, how did the researchers pick the cases (the patients with the disease or outcome of interest), and how did they pick the people who act as the controls? Given that the researchers are looking for cases with a specific disease, they should report clearly how they have defined that disease and by what criteria they have measured it.

The populations that both groups of patients are drawn from should be similar; if there are significant differences, you should ask why and if this might be a significant confounding factor in the differences in exposures that both groups might had had in the past.

The effect of confounding factors and how controls are selected is one of the more controversial parts of case control studies; remember that unlike in a randomized controlled trial (RCT), sampling is not random. The method by which controls are selected results in case control studies being defined in one of two ways: matched or unmatched. In unmatched studies, the researchers will enrol controls without worrying about the number they enrol or the confounding factors that they might have. The controls should come from a population similar to that of the cases, but beyond that little screening of the background of the controls is done. The problem is that, as described, the selection pays no attention to the possible effect of confounders, and the way to try to address this is to match the controls to the cases. In matched case control studies, the controls are enrolled based on a factor that the researchers might think is a confounder, a good example being sex of the patient. In an unmatched case control study, no regard would be paid to the sex of the controls or the cases during enrolment, but in a study matched for sex the enrolment would ensure that there was the same split between the sexes within each group. As such, sex can be removed as a potential confounder.

There are two types of matched case control studies: matching where a case is matched to a set number of controls (based on one or more confounding factors) and matching where the overall frequency of a confounder is kept the same between the groups (as described earlier, 'frequency matching').

Not all patients approached, in both the case and control groups, will be willing to participate. You should look at the rates of participation in each group. If there are differences, ask if this might indicate a difference in the populations the cases and controls are being drawn from, or that the researchers are approaching potential cases and controls differently. If either of these is true, there is potential bias in the study result.

How Did the Researchers Define the Disease?

How the disease that is being studied is defined is clearly important. If the researchers are looking to study people with hypertension, what definition of hypertension have they used, is this justifiable and how have they ensured the patients meet that definition? Equally, you must be sure that the control patients do not have the disease; how have the researchers ensured this? Looking at a situation where the researchers are looking into patients with hypertension, it is easy to see how easily patients with undiagnosed hypertension might be enrolled as controls if the researchers only used general practitioner (GP) records of the presence or lack of a diagnosis of hypertension.

Did the Researchers Know What the Participants Were Exposed to before They Started?

In case control studies, the researchers will look back in time to look at what exposures the cases and controls had and try to draw conclusions from this. In order that selection of participants for a trial is done in an unbiased way, efforts should be made to demonstrate to the reader that the researchers were unaware of the exposure status of people before they were enrolled.

The relevant factors about the exposure (such as timing, length of exposure and quantity) should be recorded for both groups, and the method for questioning and recording this should be the same for participants in both groups. Again, if there are differences in the way information is gathered between the groups, question why and consider that the results may be affected by bias.

Cohort Studies

When considering the methodology of cohort studies, there is a lot of overlap with the way in which we critically appraise randomized controlled trials; we need to consider how the patients were selected to be analyzed in each group and whether any difference observed between the two groups is likely to be solely due to the difference in treatment they were observed to received. (Please note that in the case of cohort studies the 'treatment' is used to describe the area of interest being investigated such as risk factor.)

Who Did They Include and Did They All Make It to the End?

As in case control studies, consider how the researchers picked the patients who they analyzed in the cohort group. Did they convince you that they included all the patients who received the intervention of interest? If they excluded some, why was that and could they be 'cherry-picking' the best cases? For the cohort of patients they compared with, how did they select them? Are they from a similar population with the same disease and of a similar severity? The inclusion and exclusion criteria for patients should be the same in both groups.

Because, by definition, cohort studies are not randomized, there is no intrinsic mechanism to ensure that confounding factors will be spread equally between the two groups. As a result, you should consider the factors that you think might act as confounders and check that they have both been recorded (at baseline and ideally during the course of the study) and that they are equally spread between the two groups; the researchers should have made efforts to ensure this, and this should be clear to you.

Finally, with regard to who the researchers enrolled, consider if both groups were followed up for the same length of time. Given that diseases will usually progress over time (and more people will die over time), unequal length of follow-up would represent a significant bias. Look to see if the dropout rate varies between the groups, both the total number of dropouts and the rate at which they dropped out. Although some patients dropping out from a trial is considered normal (and a very low or no dropout rate in a prospective trial is somewhat suspicious in itself), if there are significant differences in dropouts between groups, consider whether this might suggest systematic differences between them that might mean the two groups are not truly comparable.

Were Both Groups Treated the Same?

You must be convinced that the only difference between the two groups is the intervention being given or not given or the risk factor of interest being present or not. If there are other treatment differences, it is possible that it is those, rather than the intervention, that has resulted in any differences in outcome. Because cohort studies are often not as tightly managed as randomized controlled trials, there are often differences in the treatment that the two groups receive. This is particularly true if the control group is a historical control or from a different hospital or geographical area. Remember, we know that outcomes vary between treatment centres, and indeed we expect outcomes to improve as medical care advances over time, so use of a control group from the past or a different place will make the result less reliable.

Did the Researchers Know What Happened to the Patients before They Started the Study?

Cohort studies can be prospective or retrospective. Naturally in truly prospective studies, it is impossible for the researchers to know what will happen to the patients they enrol; they simply enrol them and then record what happens. However, where researchers are going back to pull data from a database that has already been created, it would be possible that they could know what had happened to the patients (e.g. did they survive or not?) before they make the decision about whether to include them in the trial. If the researchers have not protected against this, the decision about whether to include patients may be influenced by this information, and hence the result influenced by bias.

Cross-Sectional Studies and Ecological Studies

Who Did They Include?

The researchers will have tried to take a snapshot of people from a population. As such, the population they have chosen should be clearly defined and explained, including from where geographically the patients were selected. The eligibility criteria that they have used should be explicitly stated, and how they went about approaching them should be explained. In ecological studies the data sources used and the rationale for picking them should be explained.

What Did They Look At?

The researchers should make clear all the variables (disease, exposures, how many and how defined) that they have collected. They should have decided this before they started the trial, demonstrate the methods how this was done and then report on these in the results. They should have a system for assessing the risk of bias and a method for dealing with this.

RESULTS

Case Control Studies

In case control studies, we are looking at patients who have the disease and comparing them in terms of what risks they have been exposed to in the past with patients who do not have the disease. As we described in the methods section earlier, the study may be matched or unmatched, and this must be stated by the researchers and an appropriate statistical analysis done to account for that.

The authors should be able to provide an estimate of risk and hence generate a p-value and confidence interval. The same rules that we have described previously apply; ideally, authors should publish both a p-value and confidence interval for the results, but we find the confidence interval more useful.

Cohort Studies

Just as we described in the methods section earlier that there is a lot of crossover between the way we can think about cohort studies and RCTs, this is also true of the results. In a cohort study, just as in an RCT, we are looking at the effect a difference in treatment might have on outcome, and thus essentially we are comparing the rates of the outcome (be it death, length of hospital stay or something else) between the groups. Just as with an RCT, we can calculate the risk in the group that received the intervention (or risk factor) that we are interested in and the risk in those that did not. Similarly, we can compare the risk in the two groups by dividing the risk in the group with the intervention by the risk in the group without the intervention – calculating a relative risk just as we would with an RCT.

The calculations and theory behind this are covered in Chapter 8 on therapeutic studies.

Cross-Sectional and Ecological Studies

Given that these studies are looking at a single point in time, the results section should cover the estimate for the data they were looking for (and which should have been explained fully in the design and methods sections). A lot of data can be collected in a cross-sectional study, about both disease and exposure to risk factors, and the authors should provide results for all the data they set out to collect. The authors should calculate an unadjusted value for each data set, but in an ideal world, they should have also taken into account confounders and other biases and they should provide us with a second result adjusted for these factors. Importantly, while it is understandable to provide an unadjusted but not adjusted result, we would argue strongly that if the authors only provide an adjusted result, this should raise concerns.

CONCLUSIONS

Because of the nature of observational trials, it is generally regarded as impossible to judge *causation* from them; rather, different strengths of *correlation* might be shown. When trying to assess the degree of correlation between an exposure or risk factor and an outcome and whether this is likely to be a causative relationship, classically we use a set of criteria first described by Sir Austin Bradford Hill, a British epidemiologist, in 1965. The more criteria present, the greater the chance that causation is present (but never 100% certain). These are:

1. *Strength of the association* (the stronger the association, the greater the chance of causation)
2. *Consistency* (if the result can be reproduced by different people at different times)
3. *Specificity* (the idea that an exposure leads to one disease)
4. *Temporality* (the disease must occur after the exposure)
5. *Biological gradient* (e.g. the more you smoke, the greater your chance of lung cancer)
6. *Plausibility* (the link between the exposure and the disease ought to make scientific sense, although bear in mind that medical science evolves and changes its opinion regularly)
7. *Coherence* (knowledge of the natural history of the disease and of the effects of any exposure must be consistent with a causative relationship)
8. *Experiment* (if we remove the exposure, does the disease stop occurring (or reduce in frequency)
9. *Analogy* (looking for evidence from other examples that we can draw from to help us decide if there is a causative relationship, e.g. looking at the example of smoking and lung cancer to help us decide about passive smoking and lung cancer)

When reading a study, it is always important that you explicitly form your own conclusion from your interpretation of the internal validity of the trial – do you think it was well designed and run to answer the question that was being asked, and what is your interpretation of the answer provided by the results? Consider the Bradford Hill criteria and try to form an opinion about where any relationships between exposures and risk factors might be causative. Once you have done this, it is possible to compare what you would have concluded from the trial with what the authors have concluded – if those two things are different, consider why that might be and whether you or the authors can truly explain the position taken.

Take-Home Message

1. Observational trial are where the researchers do not influence what happens to the patients and merely record risk factors, exposure to treatments or drugs and outcomes.
2. Be wary of studies that are re-using data sets due to the risk of false positive results (type 1 error).
3. Many of the rules we use for interventional trial critical analysis can be applied to observational trials, particularly considering strengths and weaknesses of internal and external validity.
4. When trying to decide if a relationship (correlation) seen in an observational trial might be causative, consider the Bradford Hill criteria.

7 Qualitative Papers

In this chapter, we look at what qualitative research is, why it is done, the different methodologies, the ethical considerations and how to appraise qualitative papers.

WHAT IS QUALITATIVE RESEARCH?

Qualitative research is a type of research used to understand experience, feelings, perspectives and beliefs. It is used to explore issues when there is little knowledge about a subject and when we want to understand phenomena, the experiences and attitudes of individuals or communities. It enables us to understand and interpret information (data) that is not in a numerical format. This non-numerical data generally, but not always, is generated through observing situations and by what people tell us.

Before we look into appraising qualitative papers, we need to look at three key questions:

1. Why do qualitative research?
2. What are the different methods of qualitative research?
3. What are the ethical considerations of qualitative research?

WHY DO WE NEED QUALITATIVE RESEARCH?

Qualitative research is really important when we want to understand the experiences of individuals and communities.

It enables us to ask questions like: Why does this happen? What do you think about this? What are your experiences of …? How does it feel to be …?

It is important that this is different to quantitative research, when we typically ask questions like: How many? How much?

Example: How to Understand Waiting Times for an Operation

Quantitative Research	Qualitative Research
How many people are waiting?	What are the experiences of people who are waiting for an operation?
What are the demographics of this group?	How do people feel about waiting for an operation?
How long do they wait?	What does 'recovery' mean to those who have had the operation?
What is the effect of waiting on length of stay?	What are other people's experiences and what does that tell us?
What is the effect of waiting on recovery times?	
How does this compare with other types of surgery?	

In this example, the type of research that is undertaken will produce different perspectives, but both have come from the same question. When you are deciding which type of research to use, or appraising a qualitative paper, think carefully about the purpose of the research. What type of information did the author need to know in order to answer the question?

Example: Sunday Lunch Phenomenon

Do you like Sunday lunch? This is a relatively simple question which means all sorts of things to different people.

Sunday lunch to me is roast beef and trimmings at my mum's house, but Sunday lunch to my friend Sarah is a lazy big brunch with her boyfriend in a restaurant in Brighton. Sunday lunch to my friend Dave, who works at a nursing home on weekends, is spent eating a sandwich in the staff coffee room. Each of us has different experiences of Sunday lunch, so if you ask us all the same question, 'Do you like Sunday lunch?' our answers will be specific to our own experiences and the different things we understand to mean 'Sunday lunch'. So, in this situation, simple yes and no answers do not tell us anything very useful.

Instead, if we used qualitative research to answer this question, we could ask: What is your experience of Sunday lunch? How does it make you feel? How does Sarah's experiences compare with Dave's? How do they both compare with mine? What are the common themes about Sunday lunch that mean the same to us all, and what are the differences? Why is there a difference?

DIFFERENT TYPES OF QUALITATIVE RESEARCH

Just as there are different types of methodology for quantitative research, there are also different types of qualitative methodology.

When appraising qualitative papers, ask yourself whether the researcher used the most appropriate methodology to answer the research question. They need to ask themselves:

- What is already known about this subject?
- Where has this knowledge come from?
- What did the author want to discover?
- Where did this new information come from?

When you have analyzed the literature review within the paper, you should be able to start looking at the methodology.

There are many different types of methodology for qualitative research, and it is important to understand the differences. Each one looks at the process of understanding the research question in a different way and from a different perspective.

Understanding why a specific methodology was selected is important. Research findings can be different depending on how and why specific data was acquired and analyzed. Ask yourself, did the author use the best methodology to address the research question?

Here are some examples of frequently used methodologies:

- *Ethnography:* Ethnography is a methodology often used to study people in their real-life settings. It can be used to understand how people function, interact and live within specific cultures or environments.

  For example, if a research study was developed to understand how nurses care for elderly patients in residential nursing homes, using an ethnographic methodology, you would expect the research to have taken place in the nursing home. Data would have been collected by observing nurses at work and by interviewing them in the workplace about their experiences of providing care. It should focus on the real-life experience of caring for elderly patients.
- *Grounded theory*: This is a methodology that grows theory from the analysis of the data. It examines social processes and explores the interactions and behaviours between groups. It is often used when there is little known about how groups of individuals behave. An example was a PhD study by one of the authors (E.M.) who used grounded theory to understand the role of ward sisters in the National Health Service (NHS). By undertaking long interviews with ward sisters, listening to them talk about their role and observing them at work, it was possible to understand what ward sisters thought was important about their job and how this was portrayed in reality.
- *Phenomenology*: This methodology, sometimes called the 'lived experience', explores the experiences of a particular person in relation to the subject being studied. For example, if a research study aimed to understand rehabilitation following below-knee amputation, using a phenomenological methodology, you would expect that the data would come from interviews with people who had received a below-knee amputation and used their own experiences of this to inform the research. A key component of this methodology is to ensure that the researcher undertakes the research without preconceived ideas. When analyzing phenomenological studies it is important to ask yourself whether the direction of the questioning or analysis of the data was influenced by the researcher using their own experiences to interpret those of others.
- *Mixed methods*: Sometimes a single research method may not give you the detailed information that is needed to answer the research question thoroughly, and the researcher may have decided to use more than one methodology. Mixing methods is absolutely fine as long as the researcher can explain the benefits of doing so, and how the methods can work together.

For example, if you wanted to know how effective the plastering service was in an emergency department, you might want to look at some quantitative data, such as time taken to plaster a limb, patient referral and waiting times and return rates for reapplication. However, you might also want to ask the staff how they felt about the effectiveness of the service and ask the patients about their experiences and perspectives of being given a plaster cast. This might be through a survey, or in more detail through face-to-face interviews. You could also observe the plastering service throughout the day. All these different methods of data collection would give you a view of the service from many different angles. Joining them up to form a meaningful and accurate understanding of the service would give you a much more rounded view than pure numerical data.

ETHICS IN QUALITATIVE RESEARCH

Obtaining ethics is key for all papers. But there are specific things to think about with qualitative research. When reading a paper you must be satisfied that the 'moral rules' were stuck to and thus confirm to yourself that the research performed did not cause any physical, emotional or psychological harm to the participants. Research ethics exist to protect the dignity and values of the people who take part in the research, usually patients or staff. Researchers need to recognize all ethical issues that arise in a research study design. These need to be formally acknowledged, discussed and addressed before any research can take place. When analyzing qualitative research, it is important to explore how the researcher approached the ethical issues within the study and how they were managed.

Key ethical issues include:

1. Recognizing and minimizing any risk of harm that could occur to the participant as a direct or indirect result of taking part in the study.
2. Ensuring that participants understand the purpose, benefits, risks (if any exist) or potential risks of the research and are fully informed about the study. They must formally consent to take part in the research, so these elements have to be explained in a way that the participants can understand.
3. The right to confidentiality and anonymity. Research cannot include information that will enable the individuals to be identified.
4. Explanations about the process of the research. Participants must know exactly what to expect, what will happen and how the research will be conducted. Written information is essential.
5. Participants must always be given the opportunity to withdraw from the research study at any point. How they can do this must be explained to them.

How do we know if we need ethical approval?

Some of the time, ethical issues are really obvious. For example, if you wanted to understand the experiences of young children in paediatric outpatients, it is obvious that you would need to talk to the parents and seek their permission to observe or speak to their children.

However, some issues may be more subtle and not easy to address. Take a look at the following example and think about the ethical issues you would need to address if this was your study.

Example: Ethical Dilemma

A researcher wants to understand what information teenager mothers need when they become pregnant. He wants to talk to teenage mothers about their pregnancies and ask them questions relating to childbirth.

Ethical issues include concerns around informed consent: Are teenagers legally permitted to agree to take part in research without consent from a parent or guardian? Do you need an interpreter if the teenager does not speak the same language as you do?

These issues are reasonably straightforward to address, but there are other more complex questions to answer around the safeguarding of children and vulnerable people and disclosures of information that are really relevant here. What do you do if the teenager tells you something that you deem significant to her health or well-being that requires you to inform a clinician, yet in doing so you would jeopardize her right to anonymity and confidentiality? What if your questions frighten or upset her? What do you do if she asks you for advice about choices in maternity care and delivery option? Can you help her?

So, when reading a qualitative paper, think through every detail of the study and acknowledge the ethical issues; ensure the author has addressed each of these.

APPRAISING QUALITATIVE PAPERS

Even though the appraisal of qualitative papers may not be as black and white as the science behind quantitative critical appraisal, it is just as important. Understanding how to review qualitative research requires a systematic and analytical process. It is crucial to assess the validity of the research, which in more simple terms means, did the results accurately reflect the concept being measured?

To assess the validity of a study you could ask questions such as:

- Did the researcher select the right participant group to answer the research questions?
- Did the researcher collect data in a way that would provide the best insight?
- Was the sample size appropriate to reach the conclusions drawn?
- Was the methodology choice appropriate and did the researcher explain the reasons for the choice?
- Were ethical issues acknowledged and addressed, and was consent truly informed?
- Do the conclusions drawn from the research justify the complexity of the subject under scrutiny and avoid oversimplification?
- Were the researchers' personal views self-acknowledged throughout the research, but without causing a biased or one-sided view?
- Were all possible explanations explored?
- Were findings triangulated with alternative sources?
- Were findings fed back to respondents to confirm that they reflected their experiences and beliefs accurately?
- Does this research and its findings connect with your own experiences of the subject?

Take-Home Message

1. Qualitative research is used to understand experience, feelings, perspectives and beliefs. This contrasts with quantitative research, which explores numerical data.
2. There are different types of methodology. Popular examples include ethnology, grounded theory and phenomenology.
3. Different types of methodology can be combined (including with quantitative methods) to create a mixed methodology paper.
4. Even though the appraisal of qualitative papers may not be as black and white as the science behind quantitative critical appraisal, it is just as important. Understanding how to review qualitative research requires a systematic and analytical process.

8 Therapeutic Papers

In much of clinical medicine we are interested in whether an intervention (a drug, a practical procedure, an operation, a change in process, etc.) is better than what we already do. Of course what we already do may be nothing at all or may be an older, established treatment. Trials that compare the outcomes of two or more groups that are given different interventions are termed 'therapeutic trials'.

In this chapter we work our way through various aspects of the methodology of therapeutic trials, initially with specific reference to randomized control trials (RCTs). We then discuss therapeutic studies of service delivery changes and the specific features that relate to them. We follow this with an explanation of how to understand and use the results that the authors of the trial produce. We have distilled much of this information into the checklist which is shown at the end of this chapter.

Let's start by looking at the different aspects of design and methodology of the trial that you should consider when reading an RCT.

DESIGN AND METHODOLOGY FEATURES OF RANDOMIZED CONTROL TRIALS

What Is the Intervention Being Compared Against?

In most trials we are interested in how good an intervention is, and this usually involves comparing it against another intervention, which we term the 'control' – hence the randomized *control* trial.

Our choice of control may vary depending on what we are looking at: if there is no standard treatment for us to use as a control, we may compare our intervention to no intervention at all. Approximately one in three people will report a difference in their symptoms when placed on a treatment even if that treatment has no clinical effect, and this phenomenon is known as the 'placebo effect'. Some would argue that this is why homeopathy purports to work. In order to remove this potential bias, in trials where the control group is going to receive 'no intervention', this should be disguised by using a placebo treatment for the control group.

In an ideal world the control group should run alongside the intervention group, and they should receive what would be considered the 'standard' current treatment. When you read a paper and this is not the case, you need to factor this into your assessment of the result of the study.

In some disease processes the use of a contemporaneous control group is not possible. An example of this is in rarer illnesses where it may take many years to enrol a sufficient number of people. In these cases, it might be appropriate to use historical controls – that is, compare your intervention against patients who have received the control intervention in the past. Although this is an understandable decision, we must be aware that medicine is (we hope) an improving discipline, and therefore the historical control group is usually more likely to have a poorer outcome simply due to the fact that medical care will have improved over time.

In disease processes where there is a guaranteed 100% mortality rate, it might be appropriate to not use a control group and give everyone you enrol the intervention under investigation. In this case, the moral argument will not necessarily hold true if the intervention itself has significant side effects, such as pain.

Selection of Trial Participants

Selection of participants is covered in detail in Chapter 2. The important points to remember are:

- Inclusion and exclusion criteria should be listed within the trial, and these determine which patients can be selected for the trial and which cannot.
- Too tight inclusion and too broad exclusion criteria run the risk of making the trial result hard to generalize to the rest of the population.
- Selection should be determined only by the stated inclusion or exclusion criteria; otherwise the result will be biased.
- Selection happens first, then requesting the patients' consent to enter the trial and then (in an RCT) randomization to one arm of the trial.

Allocation of Trial Participants and Randomization

Once we have selected and gained consent from the patients we are going to enrol in the trial, we need to decide which group they will to go into: intervention or control. If we are allowed to pick which patients go into which group, we will be able to influence the trial unfairly – perhaps consciously or unconsciously – by allowing certain types of patients access to one trial arm but not the other. In order to be confident that the result of the trial is a fair reflection of only the difference between the two interventions, we need to be certain that patients who are enrolled have an equal chance of being put in either of the groups. In RCTs we do this by means of two processes: concealed allocation and randomization.

Concealed allocation is the process whereby patients and researchers are unaware of what group trial subjects will end up in once they have been enrolled in the trial.

When patients agree to enter a trial, they need to be fully informed about what might happen to them. When there is more than one potential arm to the trial, what we need to avoid, however, is letting the patient know which of the treatments they are going to get. This is because the decision on whether to consent to taking part may be influenced by whether the patient feels they are likely to get a 'new and exciting' (or indeed 'experimental and scary') drug or an 'old and outdated' (or 'tried and tested') one.

This potential for bias may also influence the researchers enrolling patients into the trial, and so they too must be prevented from being aware of which group patients will be put into after enrolment into the study. This prevents the researcher from either encouraging or dissuading an individual into a particular trial arm. A good example where allocation concealment fails is when allocating people by days of the week (e.g. those that attend on a Monday go into group A and those that attend on

Tuesday go into group B). Although it gives the impression of random selection of patients, it is totally predictable and therefore does not achieve allocation concealment. Researchers enrolling patients will know which group patients will go into, and this may well affect whether they enrol certain patients.

Randomization is important as it distributes known and unknown confounders (see later) between the experimental and control groups as long as there are sufficient numbers in the study. We must not just accept that a study is randomized but should look at how randomization was performed. There are various types of randomization, some of which are described here:

- *Simple randomization* allows patients to be randomly divided between both groups. This can be performed with a coin toss, random number tables or, ideally, a computer programme.
- *Block randomization* occurs when patients are randomized in blocks. Keeping things simple, imagine you want to divide patients equally between two interventions; for each block of six patients, three would go to one arm and three would go to the other arm, but the order of the patients within the block would be random. The main aim of doing this is that it will result in more balanced numbers in each group at each time period of the trial and allow for easier interim analysis. The smaller the blocks, the higher the risk that the allocation process may be predicted and hence allow for the possibility of bias. This system can be used for any number of arms within a trial.
- *Stratified block randomization* is block randomization with stratification to take account of a confounder. For example, there is a new antibiotic to treat pneumonia, but we are worried that smoking is a confounder. We group people as smokers and non-smokers and then block randomize them within the strata of smokers and non-smokers (Figure 8.1). This will ensure an appropriate spread of smokers and non-smokers in the treatment and control groups. In trials with smaller numbers, this may not occur with simple randomization.
- *Quasi-randomization* is when there appears to be randomization, but it is not truly random, for example, randomization by day of the week.
- *Cluster randomization* is when the unit of randomization is not an individual study participant but rather a group of individuals treated in the same place or by the same person (Figure 8.2). Cluster randomization allows us to study interventions that are applied to groups rather than individuals, such as process changes like the introduction of a clinical decision unit (CDU). If we were to try having two different processes operating in the same clinical area (e.g. some patients having access to a CDU and others not), there is the potential for confusion, protocol violation and bias; cluster randomization works to avoid this. Unfortunately, cluster randomization tends to require a greater complexity of design and analysis. How this is done is beyond the level needed for practicing clinicians (rather than statisticians), but it is important that the authors tell you they have taken this into account.
- *Adaptive randomization* is a mechanism by which the probability of being randomized to a group varies dependent on previous patient allocations.

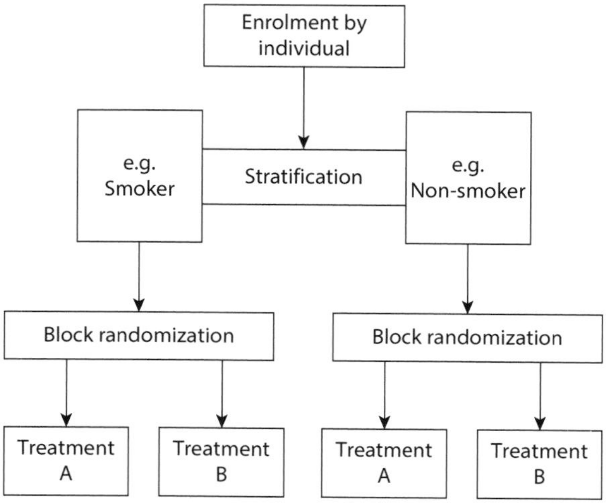

FIGURE 8.1 Stratified block randomization.

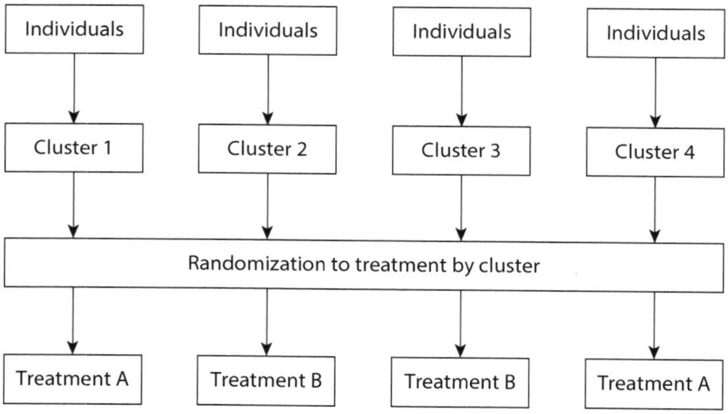

FIGURE 8.2 Cluster randomization. The number of clusters will vary depending on the study.

When discussing randomization there are several important points to be aware of:

- The more that outside influence (researchers, clinicians, patients, etc.) can alter trial allocation, the greater the chance of biasing the results of the trial.
- Randomization and trial allocation happen once the participant has been enrolled irreversibly in the trial – although the patient can decline to be involved at any point, once enrolled, the researchers should count them as having been part of the trial.
- There are various forms of randomization process, each with its pros and cons, but as a general rule, the further the researchers are kept from the randomization process, the smaller the likelihood that it will be able to be subverted (intentionally or otherwise).

Blinding

How we act is influenced by our knowledge and beliefs, and this can consciously and subconsciously introduce bias into a trial. To prevent this from happening, a process known as blinding is used. When we use blinding we prevent the people involved in the trial (e.g. researchers, patients, clinicians or statisticians) from knowing whether the patient is in the control or intervention arm of the trial. The more people who are blinded in a trial, the lower the chance of bias. There are many forms of blinding depending on who is unaware of the patient designation.

- *No blinding*: In some trials everybody knows who received the intervention and the control; this is referred to as an open trial.
- *Single blind*: Patient or researcher is blinded to whether the patient has received intervention or control.
- *Double blind*: Both patient and researcher are blinded.
- *Triple blind*: Patient, researcher and analyst are blinded.

As part of blinding, it is often necessary to camouflage the treatment the patient is receiving. Unless the intervention looks exactly the same as the control, both the patient and clinician may be able to figure out which is which, and this may introduce bias. To camouflage treatment, we may have to make the control and treatment look similar (e.g. same colour and shape tablet and same packaging). If this is not possible because the treatments are too different (e.g. an oral and an intravenous medication), a double dummy trial where the patient appears to receive both treatments can be used.

If blinding is unsuccessful, the following biases can occur:

- *Expectation bias*: Patient, carers, clinicians or researchers expect a certain outcome from a particular treatment (or in the case of the patient, based on the fact they are getting a 'new' treatment) and this influences how they experience or report their symptoms.
- *Attention bias*: Patients recognize that they are receiving a new and therefore 'special' treatment and hence are receiving greater attention than normal, which makes them more likely to interpret their situation more positively.

The difference between allocation concealment and blinding is an important one, and it is important that you understand that allocation concealment occurs in order to prevent people from knowing what trial group participants *will* go into, whereas blinding prevents people knowing which group they are in *once they are in the trial* (Figure 8.3).

Although in the ideal world all people involved in a trial should be blind to the intervention each patient has received, this is not always possible. For example, the past few years have seen a number of papers on cooling post–cardiac arrest survivors. Given that those in the intervention group needed to have their temperature maintained at a particular level, those providing the intervention needed to

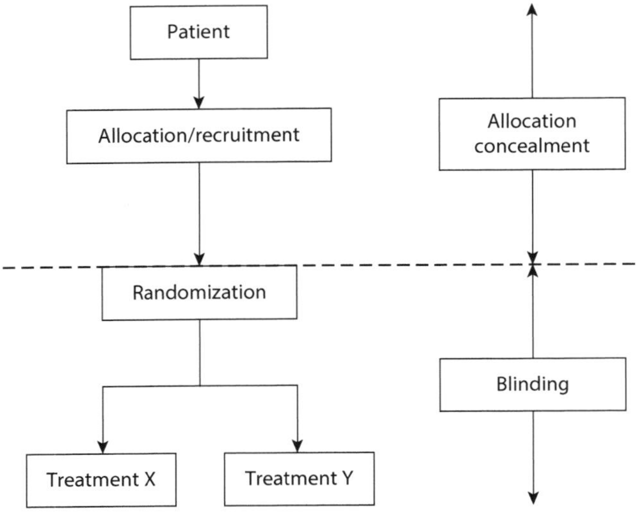

FIGURE 8.3 Many clinicians struggle with the difference between allocation concealment and blinding. Allocation concealment is used to prevent bias up to the point of randomization, whereas blinding is used after randomization.

know who was in each group. This does not, however, mean that no blinding can happen at all. For example, the people interpreting the results from the patients, including analyzing clinical outcome, can still be blinded to what treatment group each patient was in.

As a final point, it is worth mentioning that in some cases, a lack of blinding may be more likely to cause problems than others. When measuring outcomes such as 'died or did not die', the interpretation is less prone (although not immune) to bias than when recording outcomes such as patient satisfaction, where a degree of interpretation of the answer from the patient may be possible.

Were All the Patients Accounted For?

Once enrolled in the study (which includes gaining the patient's consent), the patient becomes irreversibly part of the study. Of course, the patient may or may not complete the study as planned. This may be for a variety of reasons, including protocol violation (e.g. due to physician choice or intolerability of the intervention) or being lost to follow-up. This is to be expected in a proportion of the trial participants and should be planned for when the sample size is being calculated. However, a good RCT should record and publish how the patients flowed through the trial and what happened to the patients who for whatever reason either failed to get enrolled in the first place or did not reach the end of the trial.

International guidance, the Consolidated Standards of Reporting Trials (CONSORT) statement 2010, tells researchers the recommended format for reporting their trial. As part of this, RCTs should produce a flow chart showing what

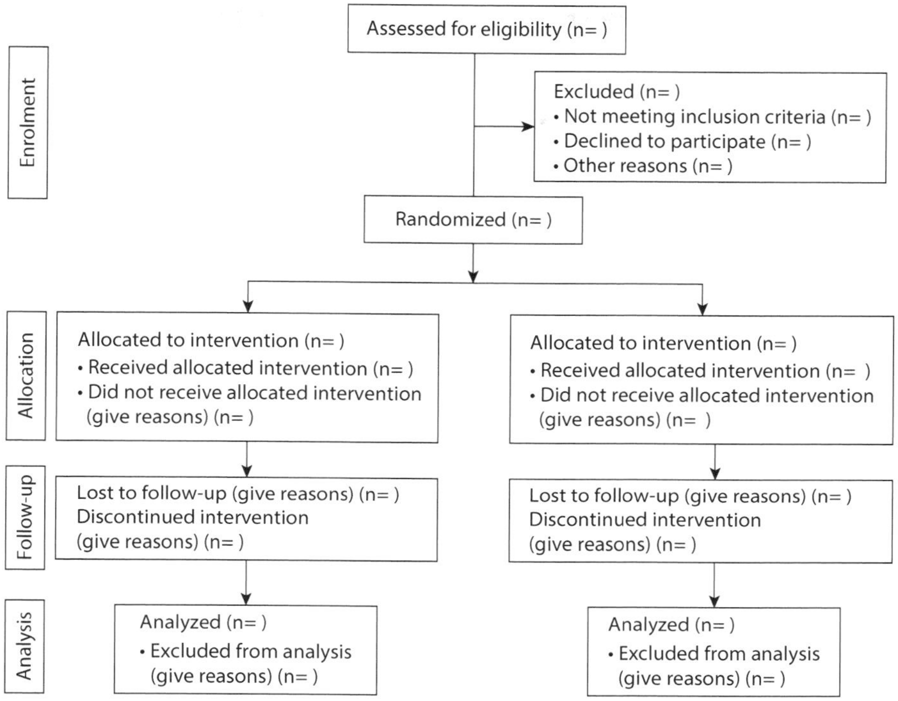

FIGURE 8.4 CONSORT flow diagram.

happened to all the patients in the study and how many had their results analyzed. It is usually the first diagram in a study and is labelled the CONSORT flow diagram, an example of which is given in Figure 8.4.

Once you have looked at the CONSORT flow diagram, consider whether the amount of patients successfully followed up seems appropriate. It is reasonable to expect some patients to be lost to follow-up, but the acceptable rate will vary depending on the outcome that is being measured. For example, we would expect a low rate if the study is looking at in-hospital mortality, as this data should be relatively easy to track down, whereas an outcome measured by postal follow-up is likely to result in far greater loss to follow-up.

What Sort of Outcome Did They Look At?

The aim of most trials is to look at an intervention and see what it does. As clinicians we are most interested in whether an intervention makes people better, but how do we measure that? If we think about a trial comparing two antihypertensives, what is 'better'? Perhaps it is a lower rate of cardiac disease or stroke, perhaps it is the one with the least side effects or perhaps it is something else. We divide outcomes into two main groups: clinical end points and surrogate end points.

Clinical End Points

Clinical end points are features that are important to the patient and as such are the outcomes that measure how the patients feel or cope or how likely they are to survive or develop a certain disease.

Outcomes such as death or the rate at which people develop a disease are conceptually easy to understand and their measurement, if done properly, should be reliable. They are usually termed 'hard clinical end points'. It may take a long time for these outcomes to happen, and therefore it may cost a lot to run the trial, meaning that not infrequently they are not reported by trials.

Measures of how the patient feels or assessments of their quality of life are often referred to as 'soft clinical end points', and because they may be prone to interpreter and reporter bias, many people are instinctively wary of them. When measuring outcomes that may be seen to be open to these sorts of bias, it is important that the researchers use a scoring system that has been properly validated and which has the effect of making them slightly less 'soft'.

The *primary end point* is the main parameter of interest. It is the outcome that is used to calculate the sample size and for which a study is powered.

Secondary end points are parameters that are measured as part of the study but that the study is not designed to look at specifically. As such they may be interesting, but the results of a secondary outcome should not be used as definitive evidence since the study is not powered to look at them.

Composite end points are combinations of outcome measures, for example, all cardiovascular deaths rather than strokes or myocardial infarctions individually.

Surrogate End Points

Surrogate end points are usually factors such as laboratory test results that can often be obtained relatively quickly and easily. With these sorts of outcomes, the researchers are suggesting that a change in the surrogate end point (e.g. blood pressure) equates to a clinical end point (e.g. a reduction in the risk of stroke). Surrogate end points, given that they are by definition not the actual things that patients are interested in, should be viewed with a degree of caution. Certainly if we are to accept that a reduction in a surrogate outcome is important, we need to be convinced of the clinical argument that changes in the surrogate lead consistently to changes in the clinical outcomes that we are interested in.

Look for Confounders

Confounding is different to bias, which we discussed in Chapter 2. It is an error in interpretation of the meaning of the study result, and as such the results may be accurate and precise, but false conclusions are drawn due to assuming the different groups are the same in every way except the intervention. Confounders are extraneous factors which can affect the outcome and will lead to invalid inferences if not distributed equally or taken into account. They may be positive (inferring an association when not really present) or negative (hiding an association which is present). Common confounders in most medical trials are age, gender, smoking and socioeconomic group.

Before we look at the result we need to ask ourselves whether there are any differences between the two groups that may have influenced the result. Any random method of sampling may simply, due to chance, result in there being differences between the groups that are beyond the control of the researchers. Good-quality randomization of sufficiently large numbers of patients will reduce this, but there is always a chance that it will happen, and if it does, we need to take that into account when assessing the result of the trial. These differences could be 'confounding factors'.

Interventional trials should provide a table showing the baseline characteristics of the different groups, and this is usually labelled 'Table 1' in most papers. When reading a trial, we need to check this table to see if we pick up any differences that we think might be important. In some trials, the authors will help by providing results of tests of the hypothesis (p-value) to try to tell us whether any difference between the groups is statistically significant.

Although the table we have described will report the baseline characteristics that the authors have collected, we cannot rely on the fact that they will have considered or collected every confounding factor. Imagine our trial comparing one antihypertensive against another looking at the rate of stroke at 6 months; we collect data about the age, sex and body mass index and present that in the paper that we publish. If, however, we had not thought to collect data about whether patients smoke, it is possible that one group might have significantly more smokers than the other, and it is obvious that this may well have a large impact on the outcome (stroke) that we are interested in. As such smoking would be classed as an 'unknown confounder'. Although the confounder is unknown in this case, it is obvious that it should have occurred to us and we would list this as one of our critiques of the paper. With other less obvious confounders, we might not notice this, however. The purpose of randomization is that it acts to spread the confounders that we know, the ones we can guess about and the ones we do not know, evenly between the groups.

Confounders can be controlled by means of:

- Good study design
- Randomization if there are sufficient patients in the study
- If confounders are known, then they can be adjusted for in an analysis

If the confounder is known prior to study design, then the study design can:

- Restrict it (e.g. avoiding respiratory arrests that are more likely to be pulseless electrical activity [PEA] or asystolic in cooling studies).
- Allocate by minimization. This is a process whereby instead of patients being allocated to treatment groups purely by a random process, we control the allocation to ensure equal numbers of confounders are put in each of the treatment arms. This can be pure minimization where there is no randomization or by randomization that is weighted by a confounding factor – the mechanics of this process do not need to be known and understood by clinicians, as opposed to statisticians and study designers, who do need to understand this.
- Match confounders so that there are equal numbers of confounders in each group – stratified randomization.

Confounders can be controlled during the analysis:

- Standardization: Risk in the exposed group is calculated as if the confounder was the same, for example, adjusted hospital mortality by age.
- Stratified by separating the data into groups (or strata) based on the confounder.
- Multivariate analysis, which takes into consideration more than one confounder.

How Did They Analyze Their Results?

Consider having a trial with two groups of patients: one randomized to the intervention and one to the control. Once patients have been enrolled into the trial, we have talked about the fact that they must be accounted for in the CONSORT flow diagram. We have also mentioned that not all the patients allocated to a group will complete the treatment that they were allocated to.

There are two main ways of dealing with the fact that all the patients entered into a trial may not make it through to the end in the way that was planned: intention-to-treat analysis and per-protocol analysis.

Intention-to-Treat Analysis

In an intention-to-treat analysis, the patients are analyzed by the group they were originally enrolled to regardless of what treatment they actually received. For example, in our antihypertensive trial, it may be that a number of people who were assigned to the new antihypertensive chose to stop taking it partway through the trial due to feeling nauseated. Although they did not manage to complete the course of antihypertensive, we still use their outcomes as part of the intervention group. This has the effect of lessening any difference that might occur between the two groups. Analyzing by intention to treat means that it is *less* likely we will show a difference if one exists (i.e. a greater chance of a type 2 error). This sort of analysis takes account of what happens in real life – that patients do not always comply with the treatments they are prescribed by clinicians – and as such is considered the best way to calculate the results from a trial.

Per-Protocol Analysis

Per-protocol analysis is considered the opposite of an intention-to-treat analysis. Patients are only included in the results if they managed to complete the treatment that they were allocated to. If they drop out or for any other reason do not adhere to the trial protocol, their outcomes do not get included in the statistical analysis of the results. By doing this, it might be argued that we get a 'purer' look at the actual effect of the treatment protocol versus the control intervention – after all, failure to have received the full protocolled treatment in the intervention group may not just be due to side effects or intolerability of the treatment but also because of errors of the clinicians running the trial. This form of analysis makes it more likely that the trial will demonstrate a difference if one exists (i.e. a lower chance of a type 2 error), but it may hide potential problems with the treatment that make it less likely to be tolerable by patients.

SERVICE DELIVERY THERAPEUTIC TRIALS

Most therapeutic trials that you will come across will be variations on the theme of RCT, with the variation being in the amount of blinding and the degree and type of randomization. They will compare one or more interventions – often a new drug – against a control and look at defined outcomes.

Before we move on to talk about diagnostic studies in Chapter 9, it is worth mentioning one other type of therapeutic trial and some of the features that commonly come up regarding them – service delivery therapeutic trials.

It is very much appropriate for us to want to look at how we might improve patient care by changing *the way we deliver* a service rather than simply by trying to deliver a new treatment. A relatively recent intervention is the use of an early senior assessment team in the ED with the aim of improving the speed and quality of decision making that patients receive. It is right to wonder whether the efficacy of this is something we could test in a clinical trial. Any sort of service delivery change (e.g. triage processes, educational interventions, staffing templates and facilities such as short-stay wards) like this can be assessed in a therapeutic trial that is very similar to the RCT we previously described.

Benefits of Cluster Randomization

We randomize some patients to receive early senior assessment (let's call it patient assessment team [PAT]) and a control group to receive standard care. Our next question is how we go about this randomization. The introduction of PAT is not something that lends itself easily to randomizing one patient to PAT and the next to standard care within a single ED. However, cluster randomization, discussed earlier, would be ideal for this. We could enrol a number of hospitals to our trial and randomize each hospital rather than each patient to either PAT or standard care. Service delivery evaluations lend themselves very well to cluster randomization.

Non-Randomized Sampling

Cluster randomization does, however, have drawbacks: allocation concealment is not usually possible, resulting in the potential that patients and carers will choose which hospital to visit depending on the service they are offering. Also, clustering adds challenges to the statistical analysis of the data, and the statistical power of the trial may be substantially reduced. Because of this, service delivery papers may instead use non-randomized methods of sampling, mostly by comparing the intervention group, when the service delivery change has been made, with a historical group when it has not. There are two main issues with this: First, as we hope that medical care improves over the course of time, the result may be biased to show an improvement in outcomes even if this is unrelated to the service change we are looking at. Second, if the historical control group were unaware that they were taking part in a trial but the intervention group are, the Hawthorne effect may apply unfairly to the two groups.

Hawthorne Effect

Discussion of service delivery papers would not be complete without mentioning the Hawthorne effect. In the 1920s and 1930s a series of experiments were performed in the Western Electricity Company in Chicago, the most often cited of which was an experiment where the researchers varied the intensity of light in the working environment. The results showed that productivity increased when light intensity was both increased *and* reduced. The generally accepted interpretation of this is that the act of observing a situation (including a clinical environment) improves the performance (and hence medical outcomes) of those *in all* groups within the trial. One conclusion of this is that the results obtained in research studies may be expected to be better than those that would be obtained in real life.

Generalizability and Sustainability

When assessing service delivery change studies, perhaps even more so than RCTs on pharmacological interventions, we need to be mindful of whether the change that is being suggested is something that is both generalizable to our clinical situation and we would be able to sustain. Many service delivery changes are possible within the confines of a funded and well-staffed trial but may not be so successful when exposed to the realities of the staffing template and financial environment of everyday clinical practice.

HOW TO INTERPRET THE RESULTS SECTION OF A THERAPEUTIC TRIAL

The key to understanding the results section of a therapeutic paper is drawing the 2 × 2 table (often called a contingency table). Based on the 2 × 2 table, we can then make a series of calculations. If you have an exam in this area, it is worth remembering that critical appraisal exams are about understanding what you are calculating and not just rote learning.

Prior to doing this section, make sure you have an understanding of probability (discussed in Chapter 5) and remember that in clinical research, risk is used interchangeably with probability.

$$\text{Risk} = \text{Number of times an event occurs} \div \text{Total possible events}$$

To draw the 2 × 2 table, you need to know the following:

- The number of patients in the control group who got the disease
- The number of patients in the control group who did not get the disease
- The number of patients in the experimental group who got the disease
- The number of patients in the experimental group who did not get the disease

These numbers go into the 2 × 2 table, which is traditionally written in the following way: The disease outcome is on the horizontal axis with 'positive' outcome (meaning they got the disease) on the left-hand column and 'negative' outcome (meaning they did not get the condition) on the right-hand column. The treatment or exposure to risk is on the vertical axis with being treated written above the control. An example is shown here:

		Disease Status/Outcome	
		+	–
Treatment/Exposure	+ Experimental	A	B
	– Control	C	D

In whatever format the table is drawn in the journal article, if you are trying to draw a table to calculate the figures for yourself (e.g. in an exam), we would suggest that you redraw it in the way above, as otherwise there is potential to confuse yourself, especially when stressed.

Whenever you are asked to perform a calculation from this table, always start from the definition and show your workings. It shows you understand what you are doing and will prevent you from making an error.

Calculations Based on a 2 × 2 Therapeutic Trial Table

Risk in the control group = Control event rate (CER)
= Number who had a positive outcome while having the control treatment ÷ Total number in the control group
= c/(c + d)

Risk in the experimental group = Experimental event rate (EER)
= Number who had a positive outcome while having the experimental treatment ÷ Total number in the experimental group
= a/(a + b)

From these two risks, all the other important results can be calculated.

Absolute Risk Reduction

= Simple difference in risk (outcome rate) between the two groups
= CER – EER

Advantages of ARR

The absolute risk reduction (ARR) takes the baseline event rate into account – we explain this more fully in the examples later. ARR is easy to understand. It is very straightforward to comprehend the idea of the difference in percentages between two groups. It also allows us to calculate 'number needed to treat' (NNT).

Note about baseline rate: Before we start to interpret the result of the trial, one of the first things we need to assess is how important this disease process is. Look at the rate of disease in the control group; if it is a very serious disease resulting in death, then even low rates will be of interest (and hence a small drop important). If it is a less serious disease, low rates and small absolute differences between groups may not be so important.

Number Needed to Treat/Harm

= Number of patients needed to be treated to achieve one additional good (or bad) outcome
= 1/ARR

Advantages of NNT

Like the ARR, the NNT takes the baseline event rate into account. In our opinion, it is the most useful of all the results that can be derived from a therapeutic trial to help health care professionals decide if we should use a treatment. Given that, if the paper does not quote the absolute risk reduction and the number needed to treat (or harm) – we have to ask why.

The other calculations are less easy to comprehend and more open to making treatments appear more important than they really are. Although they compare the two groups, they are not influenced by baseline rate. Drug reps often use them to promote their treatment, and so we must really understand what they are telling us.

Relative Risk

= Ratio of the risk (or outcome rate) in the experimental group ÷ Control group
= EER/CER

Relative Risk Reduction

= Difference in risk (or outcome rate) between treatment and control group ÷ Risk (or outcome rate) in control group
= (CER – EER)/CER
= ARR/CER

We must be very cautious with the relative risk reduction (RRR). Even if there is a small baseline figure for getting a bad outcome, you can show your drug is effective. See the following example.

Worked Example 8.1

NEW STENT THAT BEATS ALL OTHERS: SUPER STENT

The cardiology team has been seduced by the rep of Super Stent. The leaflet says, 'With a relative risk reduction of over 75% and costing only £10,000 more, how can you afford not to use Super Stent?' The small print says, 'Of 1000 people in the group given the standard stent, 10 people died; while in the Super Stent group of 1000 people, 2 died'. The chief executive says, 'Ok' and 'It can be paid for by cost savings on nurse bank rates'. How much will it cost to save a life? Go through the following steps.

QUESTIONS

1. Draw a 2 × 2 table
2. Calculate risk in the control group

3. Calculate risk in the experimental group
4. Calculate absolute risk reduction
5. Calculate relative risk
6. Calculate relative risk reduction
7. Calculate number needed to treat
8. Calculate the increased cost per extra life saved

Answers

1. Draw a 2 × 2 table

	Positive Outcome, Death	Negative Outcome, Alive
Super Stent (Experimental Group)	2 (a)	998 (b)
Normal Stent (Control Group)	10 (c)	990 (d)

2. Calculate risk in the control group
   = CER
   = Number who had died while having the control ÷ Total number in the control group
   = c/(c + d)
   = 10/1000 = 0.01 (1%)
3. Calculate risk in the experimental group
   = Number who had died while having the experimental treatment ÷ Total number in the experimental group
   = a/a + b
   = 2/1000
   = 0.002 (0.2%)
4. Calculate the ARR
   = Simple difference in risk (outcome rate) between the two groups
   = CER – EER
   = 0.01 – 0.002
   = 0.008
5. Calculate the relative risk (RR)
   = Ratio of the risk in the experimental group ÷ Risk in the control group
   = EER/CER
   = 0.002/0.01
   = 0.2
6. Calculate the RRR
   = Difference in outcome rate between treatment and control group ÷ Outcome rate in control group
   = (CER – EER)/CER
   = ARR/CER
   = (0.01 – 0.002)/0.01
   = 0.8 (80%)

7. Calculate the NNT
   = 1/ARR
   = 1/0.008
   = 125
8. Calculate the increased cost per extra life saved
   = NNT × Increased cost per treatment
   = 125 × 10,000
   = 1.25 million

Tell the cardiologists 'No way!' (especially not in the current economic climate).

Odds Ratios

For many people, odds are difficult to understand. As such, in therapeutic trials (although not meta-analysis) there is no reason for the results sections to contain odds of getting conditions in the control and experimental groups. There is no reason why ratios or statistical tests should be based on odds either. The authors may quote odds ratios, but beware they may exaggerate the effectiveness of a treatment. This is shown in detail in Chapter 5.

If there are odds ratios quoted, they are calculated in the way shown below. Remember to draw a 2 × 2 table and always refer back to it.

		Disease Status/Outcome	
		+	–
Treatment/Exposure	+ Experimental	A	B
	– Control	C	D

(Remember that a positive outcome in a 2 × 2 table is actually a bad outcome, e.g. death.)

The odds in the treatment group of a trial

= Number of patients who received the new intervention and had a positive outcome ÷ Number who received the new intervention and had a negative outcome
= a/b

The odds in the control group of a trial

= Number of patients who received control treatment (standard treatment) and had a positive outcome ÷ Number who received control treatment (standard treatment) and had a negative outcome
= c/d

$$\text{Odds ratio} = \frac{\text{Odds in treated group}}{\text{Odds in control group}}$$

Worked Example 8.2

ODDS FOR SUPER STENT TRIAL

Questions

Using the 2 × 2 table, work out the following:

1. Odds in the treatment group
2. Odds in the control group
3. Odds ratio

Answers

Before you start, redraw your 2 × 2 table.

	Positive Outcome, Death	Negative Outcome, Alive
Super Stent (Experimental Group)	2 (a)	998 (b)
Normal Stent (Control Group)	10 (c)	990 (d)

1. Odds in the treatment group
   = Number of patients who received Super Stent and died ÷ Number who received Super Stent and survived
   = 2:998
   = 1:499
2. Odds in the control group
   = Number of patients who received Super Stent and died ÷ Number who received Super Stent and survived
   = 10:990
   = 1:99
3. Odds ratio
   = Odds in the treatment group ÷ Odds in the control group
   = 1:499/1:99 = 0.198

(*Note*: As the outcome [death] is rare in this study, the odds ratio is similar to the relative risk, but with higher prevalence this may not always be true.)

Take-Home Message

1. Therapeutic trials compare two or more interventions.
2. Randomization is the process whereby patients have an equal chance of going into either the control or the treatment group.
3. Randomization reduces the impact of known and unknown confounders.
4. Blinding is the process whereby those involved in the trial (patients, researchers, etc.) do not know which arm of the trial the patient is in. This reduces bias.
5. The most valuable result in a therapeutic paper is the number needed to treat. This is calculated as 1 divided by absolute risk reduction.

Therapeutic Paper Checklist: What to Look for in the Paper

General Questions	Specific Questions	Answer
What sort of paper is this?	Was this looking at the results of an intervention? Was there a control group and if so, were patients randomized into each group?	
	Were the clinical question and primary hypothesis clearly stated (usually at the end of the introduction)?	
What is the internal validity?	How were the patients randomized? Was it clearly described how this was done?	
	Was adequate allocation concealment used?	
	Were subjects and investigators blinded to the treatment allocation?	
	Were treatment and control groups similar at the end of the trial (usually found in 'Table 1 – Baseline characteristics' in a good quality paper)?	
	During the trial, is the treatment under investigation the only difference between groups?	
	Was a power calculation performed?	
	Are all the patients accounted for? If not, is there an attempt to follow those lost to follow-up?	
	Were there many protocol violations? If so, was an intention-to-treat analysis performed?	
What were the results?	Did the paper have a CONSORT diagram?	
	The paper should report (or the results given should allow you to draw a contingency table and calculate):	
	Control and experimental control rate	
	Relative risk, relative risk reduction and absolute risk reduction	
	Number needed to treat (or harm)	
	Did they quote confidence intervals (CIs) and p-values? Were they significant?	
Applicability (external validity)	Are the patients in the study similar to your patients?	
	Were all relevant outcomes including likely side effects quoted?	
	Is the treatment likely to be acceptable to your patients? Do the number of dropouts from the study support this?	
	If a difference has been demonstrated, is this a clinically significant difference as well as a statistically significant difference?	
	Is the cost of the treatment likely to be worth the clinical difference demonstrated?	

9 Diagnostic Papers and Screening Papers

DIAGNOSTIC PAPERS

Studies that look at the ability of a test to predict the presence or absence of a disease are called diagnostic studies.

Diagnostic studies are a type of prospective experimental study. Often in this type of study, the researchers look to compare a new test against an established test to see how the new test performs. The test being investigated is termed the 'index' test, and the test it is compared to is called the 'reference' or 'gold' standard. However, it is worth highlighting that although a diagnostic study often uses one individual index test versus one reference test (e.g. ultrasound versus CT aortogram for looking for an abdominal aortic aneurysm [AAA]), the 'tests' used may be a combination of clinical features (e.g. hypotension, pain radiating to back, presence of pulsatile mass and over 65 years old) or an individual test with the addition of clinical features (hypotension, pain radiating to back, presence of pulsatile mass and over 65 years old *plus* ultrasound). This concept is equally applicable to the gold standard as it is to the index test.

In this chapter, we cover the aspects of the methodology necessary to assess the quality of these sorts of trials. We then move on to what should appear in the results section. We describe how the data generated by the trial is used to allow different groups of people with differing priorities to assess the value of the test being studied. The checklist at the end of this chapter is a useful guide to seeing if a diagnostic study has been conducted properly and should be thought of as a summary of this chapter.

Design and Methodology Features

When reading a diagnostic paper, closely consider the following five areas of the trial design and methodology: patient selection, the reference (or gold) standard, blinding, biases and qualities of the test.

Patient Selection

Who Were the Subjects in the Study?

As with all studies, we need to look at the environment in which the study was done and what sort of patients it was done on. If the test being investigated has been done on only children in a specialist's paediatric outpatient clinic, it is unlikely to be applicable to a GP surgery.

How Were the Patients Selected?

Next, we must ask how the researchers have selected the patients for their investigation. Is it likely that the selected sample is truly reflective of the general population, or is it possible that the selection technique has resulted in a biased sample? For example, if the researchers have only selected people who presented on Monday through Friday, perhaps these patients have particular characteristics that make them unrepresentative of patients who present at weekends.

What Was the Prevalence of Disease in the Study Sample?

If the prevalence of disease in the study sample is not similar to that in either the wider population or the population that you treat, you should be suspicious that this study may not be applicable to your practice. If the prevalence of disease in the sample is particularly high, it may suggest that it was a highly selected sample.

Reference (or Gold) Standard

What Was the Reference Standard?

The researchers need to know whether the patient actually has the diagnosis – otherwise they cannot comment on the value of the test under investigation (the index test). They should decide whether the subject has the disease by using the best test available – termed the reference or gold standard. Although we might argue that the best reference standard is a post-mortem, this is not always appropriate. As an example, if we were looking at a new test for pulmonary embolism (PE), we would want to design a trial using computed tomography pulmonary angiogram (CTPA) as our reference standard rather than using D-dimer alone.

We might use a combination of tests as our reference standard; it might be considered that CTPA plus telephone follow-up at 6 months to ensure the patient was not subsequently diagnosed with a PE would be better than CTPA alone. We must be convinced that the gold standard truly is the best mechanism available to make the diagnosis.

Was the Reference Standard Applied to All the Subjects?

Every subject in the study needs to have the reference standard test so that the index test can be compared to it. If everyone does not get the reference standard test, then bias will be introduced to the results. You might ask why everyone *would not* be given the reference standard in the study. This might occur due to failures in processing the subjects during the trial or because some of the researchers came to believe that the index test was so accurate that they did not want to expose the subjects to a reference standard that has risks (e.g. the radiation of a CTPA or indeed the cost of the test).

Was There Only One Reference Standard?

There are often side effects to an investigation, for example, the radiation dose associated with CTPA. In our D-dimer example, researchers might design a study where the reference standard for those with a positive D-dimer is CTPA, but those with a negative D-dimer receive just telephone follow-up at 6 months. Although the reasoning can be understood, it still needs to be recognized as a flaw and having introduced bias into the study.

Was the Reference Standard Independent of the Test under Investigation?

In some studies, there is a blurring of the lines between the index test and the reference standard. Knowing the result of the index test may affect the interpretation of the gold standard and vice versa.

Blinding

Who knew what? To avoid bias, all the participants involved in the trial (people conducting and interpreting the index test, people conducting and interpreting the reference standard and the patients) ought to be blinded to the results of the tests. At the least, those conducting the index test should be unaware of the results of the reference test and vice versa.

Biases Specific to Diagnostic Studies

Bias has been discussed in Chapter 2, and so we will not cover it in detail here other than to mention the types of bias that you should specifically be aware of and look out for when reading diagnostic studies. Remember that bias occurs when the trial design, method or interpretation of results is done in such a way as to build in a flaw that might influence the result. Table 9.1 reviews the various ways bias can be introduced.

TABLE 9.1
Examples of Bias in Diagnostic Studies

Type of Bias	Explanation
Workup bias	Patients with a positive index test result get one reference standard test, whereas those with a negative index test result get another, for instance, our example of a study looking at D-dimer where those with a positive D-dimer get a CTPA but those with a negative D-dimer get telephone follow-up at 6 months.
Incorporation bias	The test under investigation is incorporated into the reference test. In some situations, the reference standard may be an 'expert's' opinion. Consider deciding whether someone is medically fit for psychiatric assessment having attended the ED drunk and suicidal. We want to know whether an alcohol breath test can be used to determine medical fitness in these patients and we look to compare it against our gold standard. However, our gold standard is our current practice: clinical assessment combined with an alcohol breath test. Clearly, the alcohol breath test is both the index test and part of the gold standard.
Diagnostic review bias	This is when the results of the index test (test under investigation) are known to the person interpreting the gold standard test. This knowledge may influence the person in their interpretation of the gold standard test, for example, the radiologist knowing the D-dimer result when interpreting the CTPA.
Test review bias	The opposite of the above – the person interpreting the index test result knows the result of the gold standard.
Clinical review bias	Where those interpreting either the gold standard or index test result are allowed to know clinical information about the patient. Remember that when interpreting test results people are naturally influenced by the clinical information about the patient, including such things as age, sex, body mass index (BMI) and symptoms.

Qualities of a Test

There are three important qualities that must be assessed when looking at a test: reliability, validity and practicality.

Reliability

How Does Changing the Operator of the Test Affect the Result? We are interested in how good a test is at picking up disease, but one very important aspect of this is whether two people who use the test are likely to get the same result. If we are doing a blood test with automated machines, we would expect the result of two tests on the same sample to be the same within the given limits of the machine (which the manufacturer should state). However, where we are using a test that depends on the user's technical ability (ultrasound being a very good example), the result may not be the same between users. For example, when one person performs a scan, they might pick up an ectopic pregnancy; if it is repeated by a colleague, they may get the same result or they may not find that ectopic pregnancy. The fact that they disagree with the first person may be due to their own or their colleague's technical abilities with the ultrasound scanner (or the quality of the scanner itself). The ability of getting consistent results with a test when different people use it is called *inter-observer reliability*.

How Reliable Is the Test Done by the Same Operator? Not only is it important to know that two operators would get the same result using a test, but also it is important that if the same person repeats the test, it will consistently deliver similar (or the same) results. This is called intra-observer reliability.

What Is the Kappa? Inter-observer and intra-observer reliability are measured using the Kappa value; as clinicians, we do not need to know how to calculate it, but you should have an understanding of what different Kappa values mean and know to check that it has been calculated. See Table 9.2.

Validity

Validity is the ability of a test to accurately measure what it is supposed to measure. A valid test has to be able to show a difference if there is a difference present.

TABLE 9.2
Interpretation of Kappa Value

Kappa Value	Agreement
0	Chance agreement
0–0.2	Poor
0.2–0.4	Fair agreement
0.4–0.6	Moderate agreement
0.6–0.8	Good agreement
0.8–0.99	Very good agreement
1	Perfect

Practicality

Practicality is the ability of the test to be used in clinical practice. We must consider the economic costs, side effects and difficulty of performing the test when assessing this.

How to Use and Interpret Results

As with the results of a therapeutic study, you could be forgiven for feeling anxious about having to calculate the results yourself. However, here we show how you can do this simply, guiding you through step by step, and by the end you will have a thorough understanding of how to interpret the results of a diagnostic study.

Which Result Is for Whom?

Let's start by considering from whose perspective we are looking at the test (Figure 9.1).

The Clinician

The clinician will already have an idea about how likely a diagnosis is, based on their clinical evaluation of the patient (the history and examination). What they want the test to tell them is how much more or less likely the diagnosis is now that they can combine their clinical findings with the test result.

The Patient

The patient is only interested in the effect that the test result has on them. They will ask, 'If the test comes back as positive, how likely is it that I have the disease?' or 'If the test is negative, how confident can I be that I do not have the disease?'

The Biomedical Scientist

The biomedical scientist, the person responsible for buying the test, wants an overall assessment of how good a test is at ruling out or ruling in pathology. They need an overall answer rather than one that is applicable to one subset of the population.

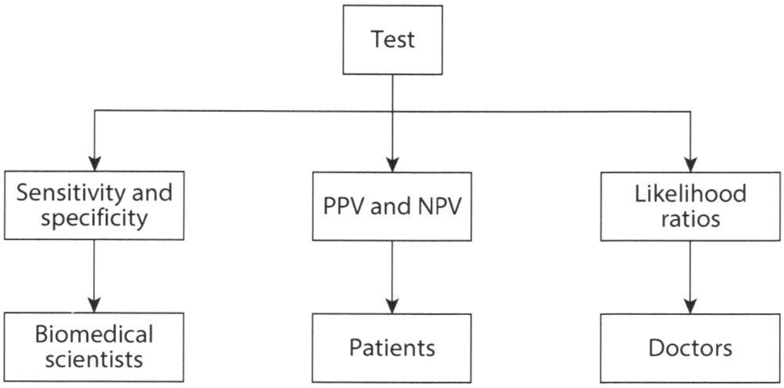

FIGURE 9.1 Different viewpoints demanding different results.

Although sensitivity and specificity are often quoted in diagnostic papers, it is clear that we also need to know the positive (PPV) and negative (NPV) predictive values and the likelihood ratios (LRs). These are surprisingly frequently not given. Therefore we need to be able to calculate them for ourselves, and this in turn makes them ideal for examiners who set various critical appraisal examinations to ask about – fortunately this is not too difficult to do.

Calculating Results from the Data

As with therapeutic trials, drawing a 2 × 2 table will be the key to understanding the results section of diagnostic papers.

Patients are classified into some simple definitions that need to be committed to memory:

- *Case positive*: Person with disease (positive reference standard)
- *Case negative*: Person without disease (negative reference standard)
- *Test positive*: Person with positive test under investigation
- *Test negative*: Person with negative test under investigation

Each patient who gets the test under investigation and the gold standard will fall into one of four categories:

- *True positive*: Positive test result and has disease (A)
- *True negative*: Negative test result and does not have disease (D)
- *False positive*: Positive test result but does not have disease (B)
- *False negative*: Negative test result but has disease (C)

The number of patients falling into each of these four categories can then be put into the 2 × 2 table. We need to have a thorough understanding of how to draw one, and remember, however it is drawn in the paper, we recommend drawing it in the way shown here.

		Gold Standard/Have the Disease	
		Disease Positive	**Disease Negative**
Index Test	Positive	A	B
	Negative	C	D

		Gold Standard/Have the Disease	
		Disease Positive	**Disease Negative**
Index Test	Positive	True positive	False positive
	Negative	False negative	True negative

Calculations Based on the 2 × 2 Table

Before doing any calculations, we need to ensure we understand what we are calculating rather than relying upon rote learning of formulae.

Prevalence From the 2 × 2 table, we can calculate the prevalence of the disease on the population examined.

Prevalence = Proportion of patients with condition (as defined by gold standard)
= (a + c) ÷ (a + b + c + d)

Sensitivity

Sensitivity = Proportion of people with the disease who test positive
= a ÷ (a + c)

A good way to think of this is as the true positive rate, that is, proportion of positive tests in people with the disease.

If you have a highly sensitive test and get negative results, it effectively rules out the condition. Many people remember this by the phrase SnOut (sensitivity rules out).

Specificity

Specificity = Proportion of people without the disease who test negative
= d ÷ (b + d)

A good way to think of this is as the true negative rate, that is, proportion of negative tests in people without the disease.

If you have a highly specific test and get a positive result, it effectively rules in the diagnosis. Many people remember this by the phrase SpIn (specificity rules in).

Remember, as a biochemical scientist, the sensitivity and specificity are what are crucial in telling you how good the test is. These results are independent of prevalence. This is key as in whatever population the test is done, the specificity and sensitivity do not change.

Positive Predictive Value

Positive predictive value = Proportion of people with a positive test who have the disease
= a ÷ (a + b)

Negative Predictive Value

Negative predictive value = Proportion of people with a negative test who do not have the disease
= d ÷ (c + d)

Sensitivity and specificity are independent of prevalence, but PPV and NPV are not. As such the PPV and NPV may significantly change if we change the population in which the test is done. For example, if a study of a new troponin test was performed on patients with chest pains presenting in primary care, it is unlikely to have the same PPV and NPV as if the study were performed on patients presenting to the emergency department. However, the sensitivity and specificity (and likelihood ratios) would still be the same.

Worked Example 9.1

NEW TROPONIN TEST

QUESTION

A new 'trop now' test has come on the market. Of 136 people who were in the study, all had trop now and all had an angiogram (gold standard). Of 33 people who had a positive angiogram, the trop now test was positive in 32 of those people. Of the 103 who had a negative angiogram, the trop now test was positive in 2 people.

Draw a 2 × 2 table and then work out prevalence, sensitivity and specificity.

		Disease (by Gold Standard)		
		Present	**Absent**	
Test	Positive	A (32)	B (2)	34
	Negative	C (1)	D (101)	102
	Total	33	103	136

ANSWER

Prevalence = Proportion of patients with condition
= (a + c) ÷ (a + b + c + d)
= 33 ÷ 136
= 0.24 (24%)

Sensitivity = Proportion of people with the disease who test positive
= a ÷ (a + c)
= 32 ÷ 33
= 0.97

Specificity = Proportion of people without the disease who test negative
= d ÷ (b + d)
= 101 ÷ 103
= 0.98

Positive predictive value = Proportion of people with a positive test who have the disease
= a ÷ (a + b)
= 32 ÷ 34
= 0.94

Negative predictive value = Proportion of people with a negative test who do not have the disease
= d ÷ (c + d)
= 101 ÷ 102
= 0.99

Earlier in this chapter we introduced two terms: true positive rate (sensitivity) and true negative rate (specificity). Before going onto likelihood ratios, we now need to introduce two new terms. These terms are not often thought about but make understanding of likelihood ratios much easier. They are false positive rate and false negative rate.

False positive rate = Proportion of positive tests in people without the disease
= $b \div (b + d)$
= $1 - \text{Specificity}$

False negative rate = Proportion of negative tests in people with the disease
= $c \div (a + c)$
= $1 - \text{Sensitivity}$

For those who are interested, we explain how false positive rate = 1 – specificity and how false negative rate = 1 – sensitivity in 'Nerd's Corner', but remember this is just for interest for those of you who are fascinated by maths – for everyone else, you do not need to understand the 'Nerd's Corner' below.

Nerd's Corner

False positive rate = 1 – Specificity
To prove this we need to prove that $b/(b + d) = 1 - d/(b + d)$.

Step 1: Multiply both sides by $(b + d)$

$$(b + d) \times [b/(d + b)] = (b + d) \times [1 - d/(b + d)]$$

Step 2: $b = b + d - d$
Step 3: $b = b$

Therefore, $b/(d + b) = 1 - d/(b + d)$.
And therefore false positive rate = 1 – specificity.

False negative rate = 1 – Sensitivity
To prove this we need to prove that $c/(c + a) = 1 - a/(a + c)$.

Step 1: Multiply both sides by $(a + c)$

$$(a + c) \times [c/(c + a)] = (a + c) \times [1 - a/(a + c)]$$

Step 2: $c = a + c - a$
Step 3: $c = c$

Therefore, $c/(c + a) = 1 - a/(a + c)$.
And therefore, false negative rate = 1 – sensitivity.

Likelihood Ratios As doctors, what we want to know is how the result of the test affects whether the patient in front of us really does have the condition. We can use likelihood ratios to help us with this. By combining a pre-test assessment (such as our clinical gestalt or a formalized scoring system such as a Well's score) with a likelihood ratio we can estimate how likely the patient in front of us is to have the condition.

Likelihood ratios can be either positive or negative. We use positive likelihood ratios when the test result is positive and negative likelihood ratios when the test result is negative.

- *Positive likelihood ratio*: How much more likely a positive test is to be found in a person with the disease compared with a positive test in someone without the disease.

  Another way to think of this is:

  True positive rate ÷ False positive rate = Sensitivity ÷ (1 – Specificity)

- *Negative likelihood ratio*: How much more likely a negative test is to be found in a person with the disease compared with a negative test in someone without the disease.

  Again, a way to think of this is:

  False negative rate ÷ True negative rate = (1 – Sensitivity) ÷ Specificity

Likelihood ratios are important tools in a diagnostic paper. They tell us how diagnostically useful a piece of information is (whether it is an examination finding, part of history or a test). Positive likelihood ratio values can be between 1 and infinity; the greater the number, the better the test. Negative likelihood ratio values can be between 0 and 1; the closer to 0, the better the test (see Table 9.3). Similar to sensitivity and specificity, likelihood ratios are independent of prevalence.

To put this in a clinical context, if we were trying to diagnose a patient with a *deep vein thrombosis* (DVT), we might use clinical assessment findings such as those in Table 9.4 to help us make our assessment. For example, having a previous DVT makes you more likely to have a DVT by a likelihood ratio of 2.5. A common

TABLE 9.3
Values for Likelihood Ratios and Their Significance

Likelihood Ratio	Significance
1	None at all
0.5–2	Little clinical significance
2–5	Moderately increases likelihood of disease, but does not rule in
0.2–0.5	Moderately decreases likelihood of disease, but does not rule out
5–10	Markedly increases likelihood of disease, may rule in
0.1–0.2	Markedly decreases likelihood of disease, may rule out
>10	Near enough rules in
<0.1	Near enough rules out

TABLE 9.4
Likelihood Ratios in a Clinical Context: Diagnosis of a DVT Based on Clinical Assessment

Feature	Likelihood Ratio of Positive Finding
Past history venous thromboembolism	2.5
Malignancy	2.6
Immobilization	1.9
Recent surgery	1.7
Difference in calf diameter	1.8
Homan's sign	1.4
Oedema	1.2

misconception is that this means that those who have had a DVT are 2.5 times more likely to now have a DVT than those that did not have one previously. Actually, what this means is that the patient is more likely to have a DVT, but how much more likely is complex, and we explain why later in this chapter.

Worked Example 9.2

CALCULATING LIKELIHOOD RATIOS

Question

Using the example of the trop now test given in Example 9.1, calculate the likelihood ratio of a positive result and the likelihood ratio of a negative result. The 2 × 2 table is shown here.

		Disease (by Gold Standard)		
		Present	**Absent**	
Test	Positive	A (32)	B (2)	34
	Negative	C (1)	D (101)	102
	Total	33	103	136

Answer

Positive Likelihood Ratio

This is how much more likely a positive test is to be found in a person with the disease compared with a positive test in someone without the disease.

$$\begin{aligned}\text{Positive likelihood ratio} &= \text{True positive rate} \div \text{False positive rate}\\ &= \text{Sensitivity} \div (1 - \text{Specificity})\\ &= (32/33)/\{1 - (101/103)\}\\ &= 0.9697/(1 - 0.9806)\\ &= 49.9\end{aligned}$$

Negative Likelihood Ratio

This is how much more likely a negative test is to be found in a person with the disease compared to a negative test in someone without the disease:

Negative likelihood ratio = False negative rate ÷ True negative rate
= (1 − Sensitivity) ÷ Specificity
= (1 − (32/33)}/(101/103)
= 0.0303/0.9806
= 0.031

Pre-Test Probabilities to Post-Test Probabilities Without placing them in a clinical context the use of likelihood ratios are limited; we generally do not perform tests randomly on patients. We assess patients and decide on their pre-test probability of having a disease. However, what we really want to know is how likely is the patient in front of me, after my clinical assessment and the test, to have the disease, that is, the post-test probability.

There are two ways of getting to the post-test probability (shown in Chapter 5). The '100%' accurate way is by using a four-step process:

1. Estimate the pre-test probability using our clinical judgement.
2. Convert pre-test probability to pre-test odds.
3. Multiply pre-test odds by the likelihood ratio to calculate post-test odds.
4. Convert post-test odds to post-test probability.

However, this is complex and is not needed. It also is not really 100% accurate as it depends on the pre-test probability, which we as clinicians *estimate* anyway. For those interested, though, how this is actually done is shown in the following 'Nerd's Corner'.

The second and simpler way is by using the likelihood ratio nomogram. The nomogram effectively creates a probability-to-odds table for us and we can use it to give us a good estimation of post-test probability.

Nerd's Corner: Calculating the Post-Test Probability Using Odds

Using the example of the trop now test given in Example 9.1, calculate the post-test probabilities for a positive or negative test for trop now for the following two clinical examples.

The formulae for converting odds to probability and vice versa are as follows:

Odds = Probability ÷ (1 − Probability)
Probability = Odds ÷ (Odds + 1)
Post-test odds = Pre-test odds × Likelihood ratio

As calculated in Example 9.2, +ve LR = 49.9 and −ve LR = 0.03.

HIGH-RISK MAN

A 65-year-old overweight diabetic smoker presents with tightening chest pain. Your clinical gestalt says he has a 95% chance of having acute coronary syndrome (ACS).

$$\begin{aligned}\text{Pre-test probability} &= 0.95\\ \text{Pre-test odds} &= 0.95 \div (1 - 0.95) = 19 = (19{:}1)\\ \text{Post-test odds} &= \text{Pre-test odds} \times \text{Likelihood ratio}\end{aligned}$$

+VE RESULTS

$$\begin{aligned}\text{Post-test odds} &= 19 \times 49.9 = 948.8 \approx (949{:}1)\\ \text{Post-test probability} &= \text{Post-test odds} \div (\text{Post-test odds} + 1)\\ &= 949 \div (949 + 1)\\ &= 0.999 = 99.9\%\end{aligned}$$

–VE RESULTS

$$\text{Post-test odds} = 19 \times 0.031 = 0.59 = (0.59{:}1)$$

$$\begin{aligned}\text{Post-test probability} &= \text{Post-test odds} \div (\text{Post-test odds} + 1)\\ &= 0.59 \div (0.59 + 1)\\ &= 0.37 = 37\%\end{aligned}$$

LOW-RISK MAN

A 20-year-old man just finished a marathon and was tired. He has a normal electrocardiogram (ECG). Your clinical gestalt says he has a 0.1% chance of having acute coronary syndrome.

$$\begin{aligned}\text{Pre-test probability} &= 0.001\\ \text{Pre-test odds} &= 0.001 \div (1 - 0.001) = 0.001001\\ \text{Post-test odds} &= \text{Pre-test odds} \times \text{Likelihood ratio}\end{aligned}$$

+VE RESULTS

$$\text{Post-test odds} = 0.001001 \times 49.9 \approx 0.05$$

$$\begin{aligned}\text{Post-test probability} &= \text{Post-test odds} \div (\text{Post-test odds} + 1)\\ &= 0.05 \div (0.05 + 1)\\ &= 0.048\\ &= 4.8\%\end{aligned}$$

–ve Results

$$\text{Post-test odds} = 0.001001 \times 0.03 = 0.00003$$

$$\begin{aligned}\text{Post-test probability} &= \text{Post-test odds} \div (\text{Post-test odds} + 1)\\ &= 0.00003 \div (0.00003 + 1)\\ &= 0.00003\\ &= 0.003\%\end{aligned}$$

Calculating Post-Test Probabilities Using the Nomogram

There are three lines in the nomogram. The left-hand line is the pre-test probability, the middle line is the likelihood ratio and the right-hand line is the post-test probability (Figure 9.2). Example 9.3 shows worked examples.

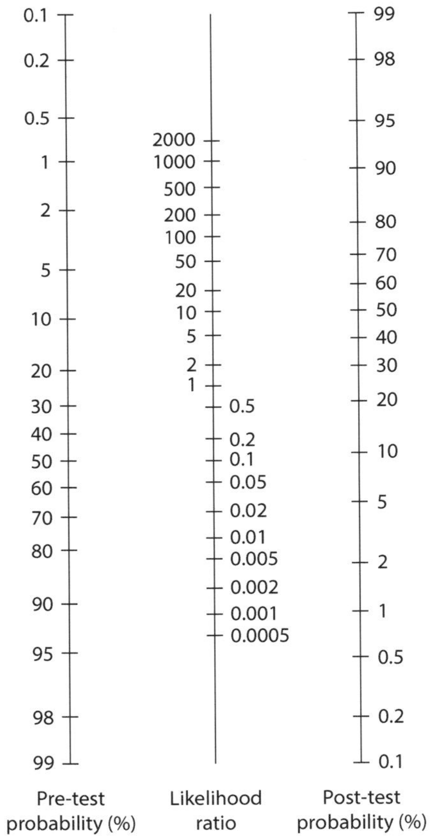

FIGURE 9.2 The nomogram for converting pre-test probabilities and likelihood ratios to post-test probabilities.

Worked Example 9.3

CALCULATING THE POST-TEST PROBABILITY USING THE NOMOGRAM

QUESTION

Using the nomogram shown in Figure 9.2, calculate the post-test probabilities for the following patients using the trop now test, which we know to have a positive likelihood ratio of 48.5 and a negative likelihood ratio of 0.03.

1. A high-risk patient (pre-test probability guestimate of 95%) with a positive test
2. A high-risk patient (pre-test probability guestimate of 95%) with a negative test
3. A low-risk patient (pre-test probability guestimate of 0.1%) with a positive test
4. A low-risk patient (pre-test probability guestimate of 0.1%) with a negative test

ANSWER

The lines are shown in Figure 9.2. The answers are all approximations based on how accurately you drew the intercepts. But they show that the answers correlate with the exact calculations.

1. >99% (Figure 9.3)
2. 36% (Figure 9.4)
3. 4.5% (Figure 9.5)
4. <0.1% (Figure 9.6)

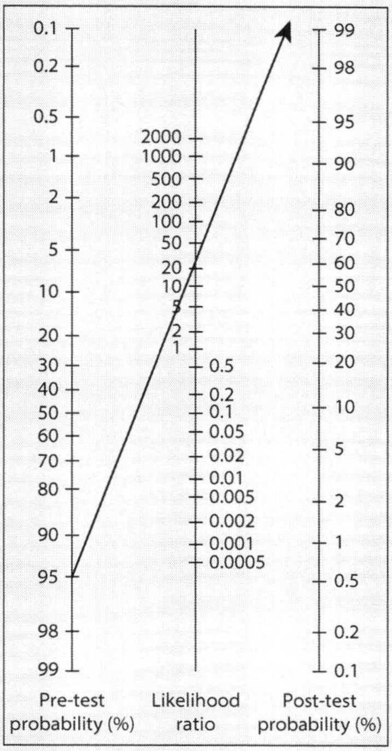

FIGURE 9.3

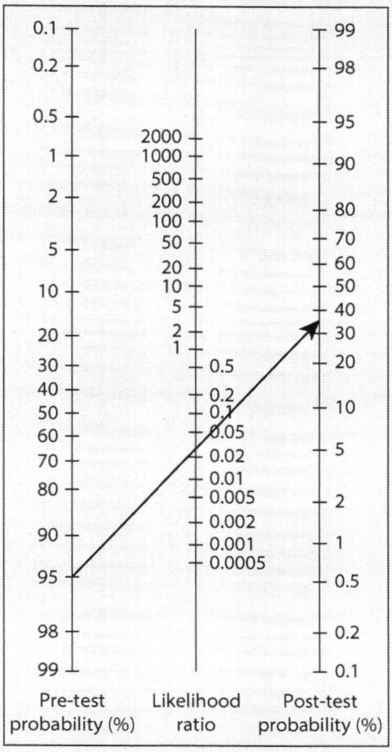

FIGURE 9.4

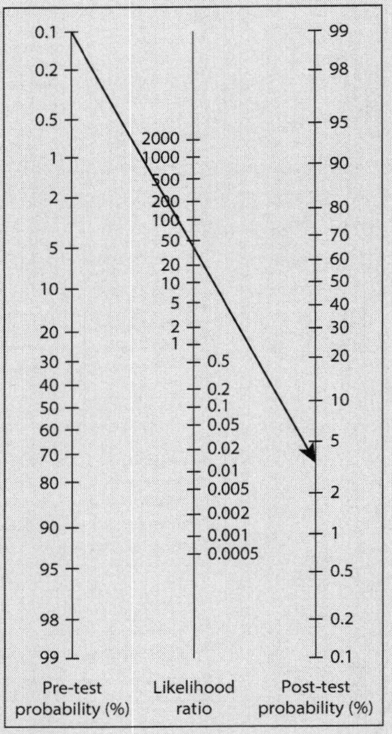

FIGURE 9.5

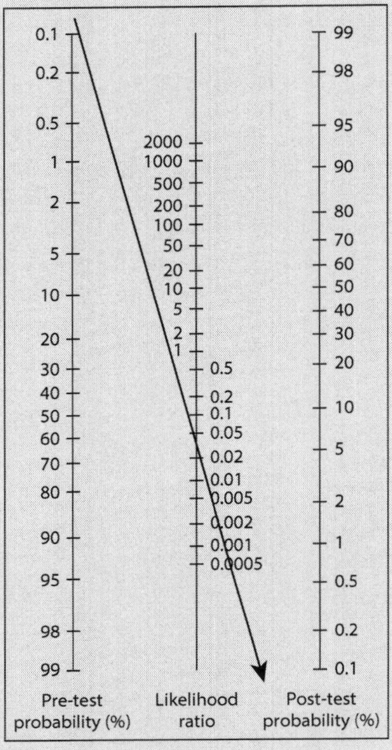

FIGURE 9.6

Before we move on, for those who want to stretch themselves it is interesting to consider the effect of pre- and post-test probabilities if we were dealing with a truly random patient; see the following 'Nerd's Corner'.

Nerd's Corner: Pre- and Post-Test Probabilities on Truly Random Patients

In reality, we evaluate patients and make our own pre-test probabilities, but what if we had a truly random patient? So using our trop now example:

		Disease (by Gold Standard)		
		Present	**Absent**	
Test	Positive	A (32)	B (2)	34
	Negative	C (1)	D (101)	102
	Total	33	103	136

Pre-test probability is the chance of the truly random patient having the condition.

$= \text{Number of patients with the condition} \div \text{Total number of patients}$
$= (a + c) \div (a + b + c + d) = \text{Prevalence}$
$= 33 \div 136$
$= 0.243$

Pre-test odds are the odds of the truly random patient having the condition.

$= \text{Number of patients with the condition} \div \text{Number of patients without the condition}$
$= (a + c) \div (b + d)$
$= 33 \div 103$
$= 0.32$
$= 0.32{:}1$

From previous calculations, LR positive is 49.9 and LR negative is 0.03.

+VE RESULTS

$$\begin{aligned}\text{Post-test odds} &= \text{Pre-test odds} \times \text{Positive LR}\\ &= 0.32 \times 49.9 = 16\\ \text{Post-test probability} &= \text{Post-test odds} \div (\text{Post-test odds} + 1)\\ &\approx 16 \div (16 + 1)\\ &= 0.94 = 94\%\\ &= \text{Positive predictive value}\end{aligned}$$

–VE RESULTS

$$\begin{aligned}\text{Post-test odds} &= \text{Pre-test odds} \times \text{Negative LR}\\ \text{Post-test odds} &= 0.32 \times 0.03 = 0.0099\\ \text{Post-test probability} &= \text{Post-test odds} \div (\text{Post-test odds} + 1)\\ &= 0.0099 \div (1 + 0.0099)\\ &= 0.01 = 1\%\\ &= 1 - \text{Negative predictive value (i.e. chance of a negative test if you do have the disease)}\end{aligned}$$

Please note, in all these calculations, roundings have been done and so your calculations may be slightly different depending on how many decimal places have been used.

ROC Curves

Some tests have a yes or no answer (e.g. does the ultrasound show a pregnancy?). Other things, such as clinical scores and assays, do not have a yes or no answer, so we need to choose a cutoff value to decide what is a positive and what is a negative result. For each different cutoff, the test will give you a different sensitivity, specificity, PPV, NPV and likelihood ratios.

To decide what the best cutoff value is, we draw a receiver operating characteristic (ROC) curve. To draw the ROC curve we plot the sensitivity (true positive rate)

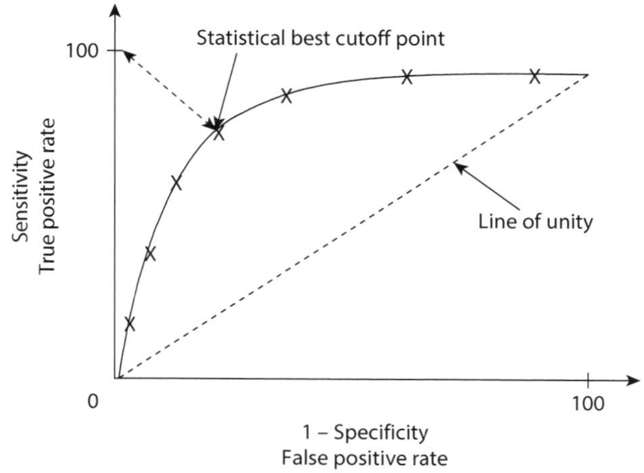

FIGURE 9.7 ROC with best statistical cutoff point.

against 1 minus the specificity (false positive rate) for all potential cutoff values of the test. The point on the curve that is diagonally closest to the maximum sensitivity is the statistically best cutoff value for the test (Figure 9.7). However, this may not be clinically the most appropriate level for the cutoff.

For example, although trop now has an optimal statistical cutoff of 17 ng/L, we may decide to not use this as our cutoff value in clinical practice. We may choose a lower value (e.g. a cutoff of 10 ng/L) as this will give us a better sensitivity (i.e. you are less likely to miss any patients with ACS), with the trade-off that this will also give us a worse specificity (i.e. more false positives and more unnecessary admissions). This will make the trop now a better rule-out test for ACS. Conversely, if we choose a higher value for trop now, it will make it a better rule-in test.

Area under the Curve (Accuracy of the Test)

The area under the curve (AOC) is a measure of how accurate the test is.

1 = Perfect

0.5 = Useless test – no better than chance and the line would lie along the line of unity

---

Take-Home Message: Diagnostic Papers

1. Diagnostic trials should compare the test under investigation to a gold standard.
2. For there to be internal validity in the study, the researchers must ensure that each patient gets the test under investigation and the gold standard.
3. If the prevalence in the study is very dissimilar to the prevalence in your population, the study will not be externally valid.

4. In any diagnostic study, the authors should state the sensitivity, specificity, PPV, NPV and likelihood ratios.
5. ROC curves help us to decide the optimal statistical cutoff value for a test. This may not be the same as the optimal clinical cutoff value.

SCREENING PAPERS

So far we have talked about diagnostic tests where we are generally applying a single test to a single patient to confirm or rule out a specific disease. In some situations, we may be interested in looking at groups of people to select those at risk of a certain disease or condition – we call this screening.

The process of screening involves applying a screening test to an asymptomatic population to define a subset of people who are at higher risk of a disease. The aim is that this subset can be further investigated to see if they actually have the disease, and those that do can be treated earlier and hopefully outcomes improved. Therefore, there are two parts for us to consider: the test that we are using and the success of the overall programme in improving patient outcomes.

A good example of a screening test is the nuchal translucency scan for trisomy 21 in the first trimester of pregnancy. Based on the result, the patient may be offered an invasive diagnostic test such as chorionic villus sampling or amniocentesis. Many diagnostic tests are invasive and may have risk attached to them, and so essentially we are balancing the benefits of earlier diagnosis and treatment against the disadvantages of unnecessary tests.

As a general rule, with diagnostic tests we are interested in them having a high specificity (the ability to rule in a disease), whereas with screening tests we would like them to have a high sensitivity (the ability to rule out a disease and hence define the people who need further investigation). When considering the screening test, we can use exactly the same critical appraisal process as when looking at a diagnostic study; we will need to consider how good the test is in making the diagnosis – that is, what are its sensitivity, specificity and predictive values as well as the costs, Kappa value and potential side effects.

The screening process as a whole can be considered an intervention applied to the population we are interested in. We are hoping that by implementing the screening programme, we will see an improvement in patient outcomes, be it mortality, quality of life or cost. It is easy to see how this corresponds to the therapeutic trials we have discussed previously. Therefore when assessing trials looking at the screening programme as a whole, we should use the same critical appraisal tools that we would use in assessing a therapeutic trial on top of the diagnostic critical appraisal elements we use when thinking solely about the actual screening test itself.

So the real question we need to think of is, does having a screening programme in a population improve the health of that population?

Thus the gold standard way of telling the impact of a screening test is to do a cluster randomized controlled trial (RCT) where screening is done in one sample of the population but not the other – and the outcomes in both are then assessed.

The reason for doing a cluster randomized trial is to try to reduce biases which you would get from looking at outcomes of patients who were diagnosed by screening and those who were diagnosed in the conventional setting when they had symptoms. The two most common biases are:

- *Length time bias*: Screening selectively picks up more slower-growing cancers with a long pre-symptomatic phase – which often have a better prognosis. Therefore if you look at the outcomes of cancers detected by screening versus cancers picked up by other standard routes, it may seem that the screening actually saves lives for that particular cancer when in fact it may not.
- *Lead time bias*: Screening picks up early disease – that is the idea of screening. Therefore, the time from diagnosis to death is increased even if patient outcome and patient lifespan are no different. Raw data may suggest that a screened patient survives longer than an unscreened patient, even when the reality is that they do not.

So be careful; do not be fooled if a paper claims that the outcome for screened patients was so much better than that for unscreened patients if there has not been an appropriate RCT to prove it. Screening seems like a panacea of virtue – but always keep a suspicious mind.

Nerd's Corner

Thinking about the impact of a screening test on a population helps us to rethink some concepts about diagnostic tests.

Screening papers should look at the impact of the test on outcome and not be just about the test itself. Should the same hold true for diagnostic papers?

Diagnostic studies have always traditionally been about how good a new test is at picking up the condition of interest. But as clinicians, we are actually more interested in whether being diagnosed with that condition actually makes a difference to outcome.

For example, say there was a new magnetic resonance imaging (MRI) test for diagnosing very small DVTs which came onto the market, and it was far better in terms of sensitivity and specificity than the standard ultrasound. It could pick up tiny DVTs which are often missed. Should we use it?

The answer depends on a number of things apart from how good the test is in the traditional sensitivity and specificity way. We must think about the costs and side effects of the test, the prevalence of the condition in the population and actually if getting a diagnosis improves outcome. For example, would the use of warfarin to treat these tiny DVTs actually improve outcomes?

Therefore, when appraising diagnostic papers, this is something we should always think about, which is not always commonly done.

Take-Home Message: Screening Papers

1. Screening test papers should be analyzed in two ways:
   a. How good is the test in making a diagnosis (use the same approach as for examining a diagnostic paper)
   b. The impact of the screening programme on the population outcome
2. There should also be a clustered randomized trial to see if making the diagnosis earlier via the screening tests changes outcome. This is a more accurate way than just looking at the outcome of groups diagnosed by screening and those diagnosed clinically.
3. Beware of lead time bias and length time bias.
4. The decision to implement a screening test into a population includes many other factors apart from just how 'good' the test is.

Diagnostic Paper Checklist: What to Look for in the Paper (Can Also Be Used for Screening Tests)

General Questions	Specific Questions	Answer
What sort of paper is this?	Is the paper really a study of diagnostic accuracy? Does it compare a specific diagnostic test against a gold standard? Is it a validation study looking at a previous study?	
What is the internal validity?	If a convenience sample was taken, is this really representative of the population you are interested in?	
	Do you believe the reference standard will make the diagnosis accurately?	
	Was the time between testing with the reference and index (trial) test short enough that the target condition could not have changed?	
	Did the whole sample receive both the index (trial) test and reference standard? Ensure that there were not different reference standards in use for different parts of the trial.	
	Does the test give a simple yes/no answer? If no, did they draw a ROC curve and explain how the cutoff was chosen? Is this clinically as well as statistically appropriate?	
	Was it necessary to quote a Kappa value, and if so, was it greater than 0.8?	
	Were those interpreting the reference test blinded to the index test result and vice versa?	
What were the results?	The paper should report (or the results given should allow you to draw a 2 × 2 table and calculate):	
	Sensitivity and specificity	
	Positive and negative predictive values	
	Positive and negative likelihood ratios	
	Did they quote CIs and what were they?	

Applicability (external validity)	Is the population used similar to the people you would use the test on? Did they describe how they selected them? Did they come from the same population as yours, that is, an ED with patients presenting 24 hours a day and with similar baseline characteristics? Is the index test acceptable to your patients? Is it affordable and available in your setting? Do the results suggest it is accurate enough to influence your practice?

10 Prognostic Papers

Health care professionals have three main roles – first to diagnose patients, second to know how best to treat then and third to tell patients what they think will happen to them (prognosis). To do this we need to have read *valid* papers about what happened to a similar population of patients.

Using the same methods as used in observational studies looking at harm, a cohort of patients with a condition is followed up over time to see the outcome. The prognosis is further refined by looking at subgroups as defined by variables such as age, sex and co-morbidity. If these variables do in fact affect outcome, they are called prognostic factors – and we need to assess the validity of these factors.

In randomized controlled trials (RCTs) the issue of prognosis is also invariably studied. In many ways an RCT can be viewed as two cohort prognostic studies – with the differing variable being the intervention or treatment. Therefore RCTs can also be used to inform patients of prognosis as well as pure prognostic papers.

Nerd's Corner: Difference between a Risk Factor and a Prognostic Factor

A *risk factor* is a variable which affects the likelihood of getting the disease.

A *prognostic factor* is a variable which affects prognosis once you have the disease. For example, smoking is a risk factor for lung disease but not a prognostic factor. However, renal failure is not a risk factor for getting lung disease but is a prognostic factor in the chance of survival of once you have it.

When assessing a prognostic paper, we take a similar approach to when we look at any other papers:

- What was the methodology and was it appropriate (internal validity)?
- What are the results?
- Are the results applicable to the patients we are interested in (external validity)?

METHODS

When reading a prognostic study think specifically about the following points.

Study Participants

The prognostic paper should follow a representative sample of patients over time to assess their prognosis. The key here is that the sample is actually representative of the whole population.

So, the first question to ask is, how did they recruit the patients? The best way is to get a randomized sample from the whole population; for example, this can be done from primary care records which contain information about primary care and secondary care episodes. Other ways are likely to lead to a non-representative sample and hence bias.

But studies may find this harder than going to where there are concentrations of patients. For example, if they choose their patients from patient support groups, they may get a non-representative set of patients. Similarly, if they go to tertiary centres of excellence, which see the more complex patients, then again they will have more patients with a severe form of the disease.

In addition, if the researchers choose patients based on where the patients were diagnosed, this could introduce bias. Patients presenting to an accident and emergency (A&E) department may have a more worrisome presentation than those who attend their primary care doctor and their prognosis may be worse. For example, studies looking at the long-term consequence of febrile convulsions show much higher rates of ongoing neurological epileptic problems if the studies were based in hospital than if they were population-based studies.

The sample should be representative of the disease, and so the patients naturally will be a heterogeneous mix. But they should all be put into the cohort at a standardized point of the disease (and invariably this ends up being diagnosis.)

The follow up period should be long enough to see what actually happens to the patients and also see if prognostic factors play a part. Efforts should be made so that every patient is followed up. If there are reduced numbers that are followed up, questions should be asked.

Prognostic Factors

When the study looks at prognostic factors, it must make it clear how it assessed if each patient had that factor, and this should be done on every patient. After this, the researchers must decide if there is an association between that factor and the outcome.

However, you must look to see if other variables are similar between the groups with and without the prognostic factor as otherwise you may make incorrect conclusions.

For example, in a study looking at the chance of dying from cancer and whether exercise is important, raw data may show a much better prognosis if patients exercise regularly. But that may be because the group of patients that do exercise are younger and non-smokers, and when you take age out of the equation, the impact may not be so great.

But even if this other variable is not distributed in a similar fashion across the two groups, we can perform an adjusted analysis looking at the impact of just the factor of interest, for example, the impact of exercise taking into consideration the differences of age between those that exercise regularly and those that do not.

How this calculation is done is for the statisticians to worry about – as clinicians and readers of the paper, you just need to be aware that a prognostic factor may be associated with another factor, and that has been taken into consideration before stating that this prognostic factor has an impact on survival.

However, we must always make sure that we are looking at causation and not correlation. So we have to make sure that the prognostic factor makes sense – for example, if a study showed that smoking improved outcome once patients had lung cancer, we would be right to question the biological plausibility of it. Therefore, it may be associated with another unknown confounder, such as caffeine consumption, rather than causative of the better prognosis (see Bradford Hill criteria in Chapter 6).

RESULTS

Papers may measure prognosis in many ways. These are usually split into measures of morbidity (disease progression) and mortality.

- Morbidity
  - Clinical incidents – for example, hospital admissions and length of stay
  - Quality of life scales
  - Symptom assessments
  - Disease-free survival – that is, length of time patients remain free of symptoms
  - Progression-free survival – that is, length of time in which the condition does not progress (often used in cancer studies)
- Mortality
  - Mortality rate – how many deaths over a specific time, for example, fatality 28 days after a stroke
  - Case fatality rate – proportion of deaths from the disease to number of patients with the disease over a set time period
  - Five-year survival – proportion of people alive after 5 years, often used for cancer studies
  - Median survival/mean survival length

However, none of these ways of expressing mortality are very good in explaining what happens to the whole population, and this is when survival curves can be useful (otherwise known as Kaplan–Meier curves).

These graphs are drawn by taking time periods and looking at the probability of surviving to a time point given that the patient survived the previous time points. When drawing the graph, sometimes you will notice ticks for censored data. Data can be censored because the event of interest has not been observed in some patients by the time the study ends; the patient might also have died of a cause unrelated to the disease under study. That patient's data are then censored. To have good internal validity there should be very few data lost to follow-up.

Take the survival curve shown in Figure 10.1. Two things can be calculated:

- Median survival, which is 18 months
- Survival over a specific time period, for example, 2-year survival at 15% and 1-year survival at 87%

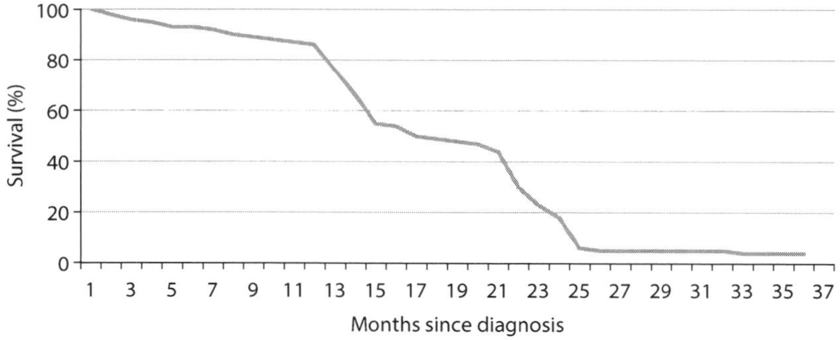

FIGURE 10.1 Survival analysis graph.

(Note that 4% look like they survive in the longer term – this may be an incredibly important thing to show to people who you have just told that you expect the average patient to die within 18 months.)

The survival curve can also be used when comparing two different groups who have had either control treatment or experimental treatment to see if the treatment does in fact improve survival. Again, knowing the statistics for this analysis is not crucial, but it is important to have an understanding that two survival curves can be compared with one another and a judgement made about whether there are statistical differences between the two.

From survival graphs with two arms we can calculate hazard ratios. These are similar to relative risks and odds ratios, but while they only look at specific points of time, hazard ratios look at risks between experimental and control arms throughout the whole time of the study. Also note that the techniques and statistics used for survival analyses do not just have to be mortality graphs – they can be used for morbidity markers, for example, time to disease progression.

Take-Home Message: Prognostic Papers

1. A prognostic factor affects survival, whereas a risk factor affects the chance of getting a specific condition.
2. The sample, from which the study was conducted, should be representative of the whole population.
3. All members of the sample should be followed up and explanations given to why there were dropouts.
4. Survival analysis graphs are much more useful than raw data, and hazard ratios can be calculated from them.

Prognostic Paper Checklist: What to Look for in the Paper

General Questions	Specific Questions	Answer
What sort of paper is this?	Is the paper really an observational prognostic paper, or is it part of an RCT looking at the impact of specific interventions?	
What is the internal validity?	How did they get the sample of patients to follow-up? Are they representative of the population?	
	What was the dropout rate? Have they explained why patients dropped out?	
	Was there blinded assessment of follow-up (important if morbidity study – less so if mortality)?	
	If looking to see if prognostic factors affect survival, have they checked to see the influence of confounders?	
What were the results?	Are appropriate outcomes measured, for example, 5-year survival rate or mean survival length?	
	Has there been a survival curve drawn, and if looking at prognostic factors, have hazard ratios been calculated?	
	Have appropriate statistics been performed? For example, what is the confidence interval for the survival analysis, and if hazard ratios have been calculated, what are the confidence intervals of these?	
Applicability (external validity)	Is the sample drawn from a population similar to the patients you look after?	
	Does this study help you give useful information to your patients (often helped by a survival analysis graph)?	

11 Economic Studies

In a world of ever-reducing resources to provide health care, the 'value for money' of the treatments and interventions we provide becomes ever more important. Because of this, an increasing number of studies are being produced analyzing the relationship between the cost of intervention and the results that it achieves.

There are generally considered to be four types of economic studies: cost minimization analysis, cost–benefit analysis, cost-effectiveness analysis and cost–consequence studies. We will review each and describe the features that should be considered when reading them. As ever, you should keep in mind internal and external validity.

COST MINIMIZATION STUDIES

Cost minimization analyses are the simplest of the economic analyses. They are used to compare the cost of two treatments for a disease (e.g. two different types of nasal packaging for epistaxis). In this sort of study they make the assumption that the outcomes from the two interventions are the same and they merely compare the cost of the two interventions.

Clearly, this is a fairly basic way to compare two interventions, and when reading these sort of analyses, you should be asking if it was possible to do another, more thorough analysis of cost and benefit and whether you agree with the assumption that the outcomes from the two treatments are the same.

COST–BENEFIT STUDIES

A slightly more complicated way of assessing the value of one treatment compared with another is to compare not only the cost of the two treatments but also the monetary costs incurred as a result of the outcome the treatments provide. For example, if we consider the recent case of the meningitis B vaccination in children in the United Kingdom, an analysis could be made for the cost of providing the vaccination to all children and the cost of providing it to none or a restricted age group of children. A further analysis could be done to judge the monetary cost of the number of people who would be expected to get the disease (in terms of health and other costs) in each group. If the monetary cost of the intervention is smaller than the monetary cost of unvaccinated children getting meningitis, an argument can be made that vaccination is the most sensible option.

Although this sort of analysis is slightly more nuanced than cost minimization, the major flaw is in how it assesses 'cost' in terms of outcomes purely in monetary terms. In diseases that do not cause any degree of pain, suffering or indeed death, this may be appropriate, but in those that do a strong argument should be made that it is not.

COST-EFFECTIVENESS STUDIES

Cost-effectiveness analyses (also called cost–utility analyses) use a different way to judge the value of an outcome from a treatment. Instead of trying to calculate the monetary value of the outcome, they use a measure of the quality or length of life the patient will get from the intervention. Most commonly this is done by calculating what is known as the quality-adjusted life years (QALY).

The QALY is a single measure designed to encompass both the additional length and the quality of life that a person might expect as a result of a particular intervention. Calculating QALYs allows clinicians and commissioners to get a feeling about the cost and impact of interventions across different diseases and patient groups. The calculation of QALY is somewhat beyond the scope of this book; however, outcomes in the domains such as mobility, pain, self-care, anxiety/depression and ability to perform usual activities can be scored. QALYs are reported on a scale of 0–1, with 0 equating to death and 1 equating to full health.

Once a QALY for the outcome of each intervention is known, a comparison can be made about the improvement in QALY versus the additional cost between treatments. In the United Kingdom, in 2016 the National Institute for Health and Care Excellence (NICE) considers that interventions that cost less than £20,000–£30,000 per QALY are cost-effective; however, this is reviewed periodically.

When reviewing these papers, bear in mind that QALYs are by no means perfect: the outcomes are not specific to individual patients, and it is well known that what represents a good outcome to one patient is different to another. Equally, QALYs do not make a good assessment of the effect of mental health and of the wider effect on a patient's family or carers.

COST–CONSEQUENCE STUDIES

In the examples above we have described the costs of outcomes in terms of financial and quality of life measures and explained that there are ways to look at each. In cost–consequence studies an intervention will result in a number of different outcomes, measured in different ways, and so the outcomes (and their different measures) are reported separately and no attempt is made to merge them into one outcome measure. Therefore, the value of different interventions can be assessed across a number of outcomes.

For example, giving aspirin in acute myocardial infarction (rather than nothing) will have a an expected outcome that we can measure in mortality, quality of life for the patient and carers and initial and ongoing costs to the health care system. We could try to merge all these together as we do with a QALY, or we could report them separately as we would in a cost–consequence study.

Take-Home Points

1. Most, if not all, interventions result in some sort of cost, and judging this against the value of the outcome is an important part of modern medicine.

2. Depending on what sort of cost you are interested in looking at, there are different sorts of cost analysis that can be performed.
3. QALYs are one way of measuring the value an intervention provides a patient in terms of length and quality of life.
4. In the United Kingdom in 2016, NICE deems interventions that cost less than £20,000–£30,000 per QALY to be cost-effective.

12 Meta-Analysis

In this chapter, we discuss different types of reviews and go through the stages of how a meta-analysis is written.

DIFFERENT TYPES OF REVIEW ARTICLES

A systematic review is a scientific study using the introduction, methods, results and discussion (IMRaD) format discussed in Chapter 2. It addresses a specific question, using existing data, and as such is *secondary* research rather than *primary* research. A *systematic* review should be an unbiased synthesis of available evidence and every effort should be made to prevent bias during the process of writing it. A meta-analysis is a specific form of systematic review with a statistical combination of the results of all the appropriate trials in the review.

The main aim of meta-analysis is to increase the precision of the estimates and hence reduce type 2 error. They do not, however, overcome bias, and care must be taken to prevent introducing new forms of bias. A common criticism of meta-analyses is that in combining the results from a number of studies with flaws, we create one big but substantially flawed study. A meta-analysis is only as good as the papers that contribute to it.

A narrative review is not a systematic review; rather, it is a broad overview of an issue. The preparation is generally not as rigorous as a systematic review; it may contain the author's opinion and only selected data may be presented. As such it may not necessarily be objective.

WRITING A META-ANALYSIS

There are four steps in creating a meta-analysis: (1) searching the literature, (2) selection of papers, (3) abstraction of data and (4) analysis. When reading a meta-analysis, you must go through the paper to see if each section was completed, as it should have been done without bias and errors and so forth. At the end of the chapter is a summary checklist of things to look for when reading the paper.

SEARCHING THE LITERATURE

When writing a meta-analysis, the first step is to perform a literature review with respect to the clinical question. As with writing a clinical topic review (CTR), a literature review should include all the common databases, relevant papers from the references of papers that have already been chosen and a review of the grey literature. Grey literature is data that is not easily available and could include unpublished studies, conference abstracts, and drug company promotional material. How and where the authors of the paper have searched must be explicitly stated.

We are always worried when reading a meta-analysis that relevant studies have not been included. This is generally not because the authors have not performed an appropriate literature review but rather because of publication bias. This occurs when the relevant studies are either not written up, submitted or accepted for publication or because they are published in an obscure journal or in a foreign language. To demonstrate the presence or absence of publication bias, a funnel plot should have been performed and presented. This is a plot showing a measure of study precision against effect size. For 'Nerd's Corner' aficionados it is worth noting that study precision is the inverse of the standard error of the result (Precision = 1 ÷ Standard error of the result).

Figure 12.1 shows an example of two funnel plots. The funnel plot should be the shape of an inverted cone (a funnel), and asymmetry suggests the presence of publication bias.

Selection of Papers

Once all the potentially relevant papers have been gathered, then the right papers need to be selected. To do this we have inclusion and exclusion criteria similar to an interventional trial. These are known as eligibility criteria and examples include statistics quoted, study design, year of study and language of the article. More than one author should perform an independent selection of papers, and discussion between the authors or use of a third author to resolve conflicts in selection is often necessary – this prevents bias. A Kappa value should be calculated to measure the agreement between the authors, and the closer this value is to 1, the better the agreement.

Abstraction of Data

Once the appropriate group of studies has been identified, the authors have to abstract the relevant data from the studies. This can lead to misinterpretation and error, so mechanisms should be put in place to identify any errors. More than one person should independently extract data from every report. Forms for data extraction should be piloted to ensure that they do not miss data or collect unneeded data. There should also be a procedure for identifying and resolving differences in the data.

In addition to gathering the appropriate data from the appropriate studies, the studies should be assessed with respect to their quality. There is no set method for this, although a formalized grading scheme is usually used, for example, the Jadad score (see the Glossary).

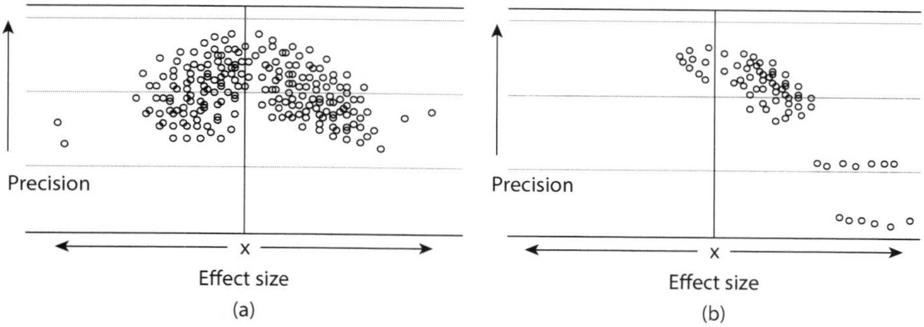

FIGURE 12.1 (a) Symmetrical funnel plot. (b) Asymmetrical funnel plot.

ANALYSIS

Analysis occurs in two stages. First, the statistic of interest is calculated for each study included. The pooled intervention effect is calculated as a weighted average of the intervention effects in each individual study. The standard error of this pooled intervention effect can be used to calculate confidence intervals (CIs) and p-values in exactly the same way we have described previously. Care must be taken to combine results that are the same, for example, odds with odds and risks with risks. The study data is often presented in the form of a forest plot (see Figure 12.2).

Even though studies in a meta-analysis are similar, there will be differences in the variability among the studies, and this is known as heterogeneity. It is measured using an I^2 value and is given as a percentage. The lower the value, the better; greater than 75% is considered significant. If the CIs of the individual studies have poor overlap, this may be a sign of heterogeneity. If a meta-analysis shows heterogeneity, then the authors must decide how best to proceed; examples of what they can do include:

- Recheck the data looking for errors
- Change the effects measure
- Exclude studies
- Explore the heterogeneity using subgroup analysis ± performing a random effects meta-analysis
- Ignore the heterogeneity
- Not do the meta-analysis

Although it is possible to combine heterogeneous studies, doing so is controversial and has a significant impact on the validity of the results.

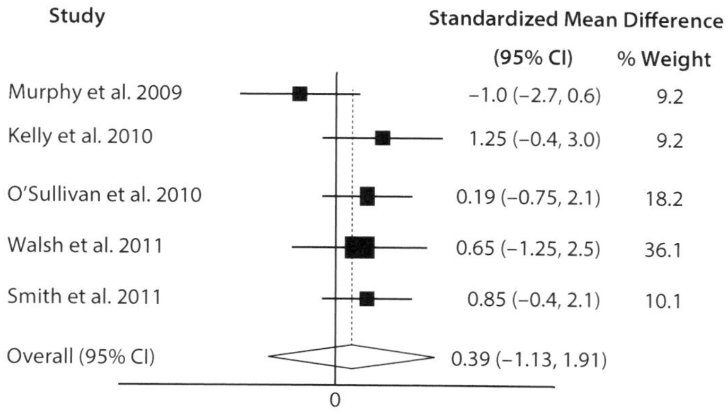

FIGURE 12.2 Forest plot. The left-hand column lists the name of the study. The right-hand column plots the measure of effect (e.g. odds ratio). The area of each square is proportional to the study weight in the meta-analysis. The lines extending from the box are the CIs. The line in the centre is the line of zero effect. The diamond is the cumulated effect, and this is extended upwards as a dotted line, which is the overall result of the meta-analysis. The lateral tips of the diamond are the CIs for the overall effect. In the example, because the CIs cross the line of zero effect, this result would be deemed non-significant.

Take-Home Message

1. A meta-analysis is a form of systematic review and as such should be evidence based using rigorous mechanisms to prevent the introduction of bias.
2. There are four steps to writing a meta-analysis: literature review, selection of papers, abstraction of data and analysis of data.
3. A funnel plot can be used to look for publication bias, and we conclude bias is present when the funnel plot is not symmetrical.
4. The results of a meta-analysis are generally presented in the form of a forest plot.

Meta-Analysis Paper Checklist: What to Look for in the Paper

General Questions	Specific Questions	Answer
What sort of paper is this?	Is the paper a meta-analysis (includes statistical combination of results from a number of trials) or a systematic review (does not)?	
What is the internal validity?	Is there an appropriate and clearly focused question?	
	Is there a description of the methodology used and have they produced a flow diagram to demonstrate paper selection?	
	Does the review collect papers that you think are relevant to the stated question?	
	Is the literature search well described? If needed, could you repeat the search based on the information given?	
	Is the literature search rigorous enough to have identified all the relevant studies?	
	Was the quality of the studies assessed and reported using a valid assessment tool, for example, the Jadad score?	
	Are there enough similarities between the papers to make combining them reasonable? Was a formal assessment of the heterogeneity between the studies made?	
What were the results?	Was a funnel plot produced, and was there any asymmetry?	
	Have the authors produced a forest plot to demonstrate their results? Is the overall result statistically significant?	
Applicability (external validity)	Did the study populations in the trials meta-analyzed reflect the population you treat?	
	Does the result represent a clinically important difference?	

Section 4

Applying the Knowledge

13 Writing a Clinical Topic Review

There are many reasons why you may want to perform an in-depth review of a topic yourself – as part of an evaluation of how you should treat patients, as part of a service improvement project, as part of the preliminary stage of a research project or if it is part of an assessment which can happen in all professions and all stages of your career. We describe these sorts of local projects as clinical topic reviews (CTRs), although if you were to subsequently submit them for publication, then they would be termed 'systematic reviews'.

Writing a clinical topic review is designed to test your ability to ask a clinical question, search the evidence, critically appraise the papers you find and synthesize the answer to your question. It formalizes something we should be doing regularly as clinicians and assesses our ability to do this. For the betterment of our patients, being able to critically assess the literature and manage patients in an evidence-based manner is essential.

CLINICAL QUESTION

A clinical question can often be broken into three parts:

1. Population (who, where, when, what is wrong with them)
2. Intervention or test
3. Outcome measure(s)

When writing a CTR, you should ask a question that is designed to interrogate the evidence-based literature and is applicable to your line of work.

Let's look at an example:

> In an adult patient with a sprained ankle is splinting equivalent to plaster in respect to pain control and fracture healing?

Another way to look at this is to divide the question into PICO:

- Population: Adult patients self-presenting to ED
- Intervention: Splinting
- Control: Plaster
- Outcome measures: Pain control and fracture healing

If you start with a root question, for example, 'In a patient with a sprained ankle is splinting equivalent to plaster?' you can then use qualifiers such as adult or paediatric patients, only studies performed in the past 10 years and so on to narrow the number of papers your search will find. Equally, you can refine the outcome measures you look for to select a specific subset of the literature.

This process allows you to generate a manageable number of papers to critically appraise for your CTR. If on your first literature review you find that you do not have enough papers, then you can widen your search terms to try to include more papers.

If you find the clinical question gives you more papers than you would like, do not throw it away yet because you may be able to qualify the number of papers in your search by using exclusion criteria, such as only including randomized controlled trials (RCTs) or not including non–English language papers. Every time you use an exclusion criterion you must be able to justify why; remember that ready availability of online translation tools has made excluding non–English language papers harder to justify.

LITERATURE REVIEW

Once you have a clinical question you can then perform a literature review. This can be done using the National Health Service (NHS) portal website or through your local medical library. Ideally, you should use more than one search engine. Examples include:

- MEDLINE/PubMed: General medicine
- AMED: Allied health professionals and complementary medicine
- BNI: British Nursing Index
- CINAHL: Nursing and allied health database
- EMBASE: General medicine and pharmacology
- PsycINFO: Psychiatry

Write your question using parentheses [()], quotation marks ("") and AND OR NOT (Table 13.1). Watch for spelling changes between American English and British English (e.g. z versus s), plural versus singular and spaces (soft-cast versus soft cast). Simple things like this can mean that you exclude potential papers and write a less impressive CTR.

TABLE 13.1
Terms to Use to Help Us Refine Literature Searches

Terms (Boolean Operators)	Meaning
AND	Retrieves results that include all the search terms.
OR	Retrieves results that include at least one of the search terms.
NOT	Excludes the retrieval of terms from your search.
*	Includes all terms with the root before; for example, fractur* will retrieve all the results for fracture, fractures, fractured and so forth
()	Most search engines work through a phrase from left to right; that is, when we search for acute MI AND smoking OR coffee drinking, the search will return all papers that contain acute MI and smoking, plus all papers that contain coffee drinking. This is not what we intended. We can force the order of search engines' process using brackets around 'smoking OR coffee drinking' to get results of papers about acute MI that also refer to smoking or coffee drinking.
""	Allows you to search for a specific phrase.

Let's consider a literature search of all the relevant databases online in respect to immobilization of ankle sprains:

Ankle sprain AND immobilization: Gives 41 results
Ankle AND (sprain OR strain) AND (immobilization OR immobilization): Gives 112 results

Now, upon reviewing of some of the titles, you notice that there are a lot of abstracts that refer to fractures, which you do not want to include. So you can change your search strategy:

Ankle AND (sprain OR strain) AND (immobilisation OR immobilization) NOT fracture*: Gives 83 results

Removing duplicates leaves you with 50 abstracts to review, a much more manageable number. Reviewing the abstracts will reduce the number of papers you have to read and critically appraise.

Remember, if there were too many papers for your CTR after going through the abstracts, you can qualify your clinical question; for example, only look at grade III ankle sprains or use certain types of papers (RCTs) or a certain grade of evidence.

It is important that you do not miss any other easy-to-access evidence, such as Cochrane reviews, BestBETs or National Institute for Health and Care Excellence (NICE) guidance. It is also worth checking for unpublished research – the National Institute for Health Research's UK trials gateway (www.ukctg.nihr.ac.uk/), the clinical trial website in the United States (https://clinicaltrials.gov/) and EudraCT for Europe (https://eudract.ema.europa.eu/). If you find any such research, you can then contact the authors and see at what stage of the process they are; this will impress the examiners and gain you extra marks.

Trying to access grey literature may also give you more potential papers. The grey literature is a broad term for anything not easily available – for example, company data and unpublished trial data. Perform a Google/Google Scholar search for your topic and make sure all the results it finds are already in your search results.

After reviewing the abstracts and titles, you will end up with a short list of studies that you need to get the full papers for. Your local library can also help with this. Make sure to give yourself time to get and review the papers. Make sure to check the bibliography of each paper you are going to include for further papers that you may not have found from your literature review.

CRITICALLY APPRAISING THE PAPERS

Once you have gathered your papers, you need to decide if the paper pertains to your clinical question. Sometimes, despite reading the title and the abstract, the paper may not actually answer the question that you are asking and as such should be excluded. Once you are happy that all the papers are relevant to your clinical question, you can begin to appraise them.

Consider using a checklist such as the ones we have provided. This will allow reproducibility of assessment and easier identification of positive and negative factors of the study design.

As part of your assessment use level of evidence or scoring systems, such as Jadad scores. This highlights that you have spent time appraising the papers. It also may allow you to exclude papers based on level of evidence if you are finding that you have too much information. Finally, it will make it easier to explain the strength of the evidence, when you are making conclusions about each of the papers.

Consider performing a basic meta-analysis if the papers are amenable to this. This would provide an excellent method of helping to come to conclusions and can be done relatively easily using software from the Internet.

Once you have gathered and critically appraised your evidence, you need to come to some conclusions. Is the evidence robust enough to say yes or no to your clinical question? Is it applicable to practice, and how would it change your practice? If it does, you need to think about how you would bring about change. If there is not enough evidence to come off the fence, how do we go about designing further research to answer the question?

WRITING THE CTR

In your introduction to your CTR, you should explain why you have chosen the topic and why it is important. You should clearly state your clinical question. You need to explain your literature search – what your search was, what databases you used, any other methods of gathering information used, how many results obtained from your search and how many papers you used. It is important to explain why you excluded papers from your finished CTR. A good way to explain much of this information is to use a flow diagram showing how papers were excluded. You need to explain your critical appraisal of the literature. You must also succinctly summarize the evidence and explain your conclusions. References and appendices should follow your conclusions. Having a librarian or a colleague check your literature search is also a good idea both prior to submission and prior to the viva.

Take-Home Message

1. CTRs are often written as part of an academic exercise. When writing a CTR, choose a topic that interests you and is relevant to your practice.
2. Refine your clinical question; broaden or narrow the search terms to get a manageable number of papers that you can critically appraise.
3. Use scoring systems when assessing the papers that you are appraising.

---

14 Running a Journal Club

No matter what field of medicine you are in, there has been an appropriate increased emphasis on evidence. As part of this trend away from 'this is how we have always done it', journal clubs have become more common. Although you would think that journal clubs have been a recent innovation for medical education, in fact journal clubs have been in existence since the 1800s.

Journal clubs provide a good and supportive way to allow us to keep up to date on the current literature in our field. They allow us to look critically at papers in a small group and make decisions as a group about potential changes to practice. They also allow us to strengthen our critical appraisal skills, and in addition, they facilitate a better understanding of research, promote research and in turn encourage better-quality research.

SETTING UP A JOURNAL CLUB

If we are considering setting up a journal club, there are many things that must be taken into account before arranging the first session. At the outset, it is important to realize that the success of the club depends primarily on attracting people and ensuring that they get an appropriate experience and hence return.

The moderator is the person who runs the sessions. This person should be interested in and committed to the success of the journal club. Initially, they should run the sessions, but as time moves on, they may be able to devolve this role to others in the group. The moderator often needs significant administrative support. The role of the administrator is to make sure that copies of the article or articles to be appraised are sent to attendees, advertise the sessions encouraging better attendance and potentially send out summaries of the discussions from the journal club and highlight any changes of practice identified. Finally, it is important that the sessions are evaluated so they can be better tailored to the attendees and hence to encourage re-attendance.

Once we have an appropriate team in place, we need to think about the goals of the journal club, as that will affect the design and logistics of the sessions. Who do we want to come? Multidisciplinary sessions allow for greater chance of introducing change into clinical practice; however, they are more difficult logistically to organize. What are our aims? Do we want to just keep up to date, or do we want to improve practice? Is the baseline critical appraisal knowledge appropriate, or should we consider adding teaching around critical appraisal as part of the sessions? Do we want to take our deliberations further – clinical guidelines or perhaps producing new research?

Once we know our goals, we can consider the design and logistics of the sessions. Should we have one journal article per session or more than one? How regularly do we want to have the sessions? How do we want to structure each session? Ideally, someone should present the paper and then give time for discussion and reflection in respect to current practice. Initially, this role should be given to the moderator. This will allow them to stimulate discussion with appropriate reflective questions, adages from their experience or by engaging other members of the group for their knowledge and experience. It also allows the moderator to assess the critical appraisal abilities of the group and to make decisions about whether there is a role for critical appraisal education as part of the sessions. Once up and running, the role of presenter can be spread to other members of the group. Do we want to use recently published articles, or do we want to structure in a critical topic review format (presenting multiple papers on the same topic)?

Once we know the general structure of the sessions, we can think about how long we need to provide for our session design. Ideally, the sessions should be maximally 60 minutes in duration, as after an hour there is a tendency to lose the concentration of the audience. Once we know the duration of the sessions we can pick the most appropriate time to run them. The time should suit those we wish to attract to the journal club. This might involve, for instance, running it as a lunchtime meeting or in the evening to provide the maximal potential attendance.

The duration of the sessions and the target audience will impact the site you choose to run the sessions. Seating the group in circle at the same eye level tends to promote interaction. Questions can be sent out to those who are attending to stimulate thought about the article or articles being appraised.

Creating a successful journal club involves attracting people to come and making the sessions interesting for the attendees so they return for further sessions. Using controversial articles is one way to do this; using classic articles that have changed management or papers which have come down on opposite sides of the clinical question may also be a useful mechanism. Setting aside a short period at the end of each session to identify potential clinical questions which the group wants to explore further is useful, as it allows the attendees to feel more involved in the running of the sessions. In addition, it might provide appropriate people with a real interest in the clinical question to present rather than the moderator. We could consider splitting people into groups to look at specific aspects of the paper and then feed their opinions back into the group.

HOW TO PICK ARTICLES

Generally, the articles come from recent journals which have articles on the area in which the group has an interest. It is often a good idea to intersperse these with articles from major medical journals such as the *Lancet*, *New England Journal of Medicine*, *BMJ*, *Nature Medicine* and *Circulation* or major surgical journals such as *Annals of Surgery*, *British Journal of Surgery*, *Journal of Neurology* and *Journal of Bone and Joint Surgery*, which may have appeal to a wider audience.

Consider picking articles which have potential to change practice or have been in the press, as this may also attract a wider audience. Checking social media as well as the papers may help to highlight articles which have created a stir and may provide the moderator with topics for conversation to help spur on the discussion. In addition, it may be worth discussing with colleagues who have been away at conferences recently about interesting articles that have been discussed in this forum.

CRITICAL APPRAISAL OF ARTICLES

This is obviously a book about critical appraisal and we have spent the previous chapters discussing mechanisms of critical appraisal. As part of that we have mentioned the use of checklists when assessing papers, and this is something that becomes useful when critically appraising articles as part of a journal club. In addition to helping the moderator to assess the papers prior to presentation, checklists may also highlight good and bad points of the paper, which can be used as topics for discussion during the journal club.

PRESENTING AT A JOURNAL CLUB

As with any other presentation, it pays to have a format to present. We suggest the following:

1. Why did you choose this paper?
2. Who wrote it, and where was it written? It is important to place this in the context of your hospital.
3. What is the clinical question asked in the paper?
4. What is the background of this clinical question?
5. Describe the study design.
6. What were the results? Were they significant?
7. What were the author's conclusions?
8. What did you think of the paper? What are the strengths and weaknesses of the design (internal validity)?
9. Will it change your management, and what will it change?
10. Open discussion to the group.

Following this format allows you to present your thoughts about a paper. It gives a basis for discussion from the group and allows people to think about how this paper may affect their management and how to go about introducing it into the clinical practice in your department. The wider the audience, the more likely change can be instigated.

Take-Home Message

1. Journal clubs have been around for many years and can be a good way to improve your knowledge and implement change in your department.
2. It requires a moderator and an administrator, but other roles can be devolved from these two essential people as the journal club attendance grows.
3. When setting up a journal club it is important to have specific aims which you hope to achieve.

15 Creating a 'Best Available' Evidence-Based Clinical Environment

In health care education we teach facts – many, many facts and probably far too many facts now that we have the Internet for quick retrieval of information. Over the course of your clinical career, half the taught facts will turn out to be wrong. The problem is we just do not know which half!

To ensure that our patients always get the best treatment, we need to continually stay up to date with our clinical practice, use social media, attend conferences, take part in Free Open Access Medical Education (FOAM) and read the literature. But most importantly, we need to do all of that while using the skills in this book to evaluate that evidence. While we believe that FOAM and social media are important in promoting continuous professional development, we feel strongly that a thorough knowledge of critical appraisal is needed to underpin this. Reading a tweet or abstract alone is not sufficient to change your practice.

Knowing how to read papers is an important skill. But what we really want to do is use the evidence we have evaluated to improve care for our patients.

So once we have read a paper and decided that we should be changing our clinical practice because it leads to better outcomes (and has economic justification), the question we need to ask is, how we do we go about implementing that change and making sure our patients continue to benefit?

This chapter looks at these two issues. The chapter then moves on to look at how we take the next step in improving clinical care – moving the evidence base forward.

IMPLEMENTING NEW CLINICAL PRACTICES

Implementing a new clinical practice is one of the hardest thing any health care worker can do but also one of the most important. 'Translational medicine' is the science of looking at how we make sure those existing treatments, which we know work, are actually implemented.

Sadly this translation from paper to patient is often performed poorly; patients get suboptimal care and money is wasted – especially on performing treatments which studies have shown are not effective. Studies have shown that in certain circumstances up to 50% of patients who would benefit from treatments do not get them. Reasons include that the treatment is not local policy, patients get misdiagnosed or human error means that the standard treatment just is not given for one reason or another.

The first step to making a change in how we treat patients is making sure you get the key local decision-makers to make it a local policy. But the harder part is making sure that once you have agreed on a new policy, that policy is actually used by the people who provide the day-to-day care.

It must be remembered that the way we manage the implementation programme has a massive bearing on how our patients are treated, and on whether they get the 'best available' evidenced-based medicine (EBM) and thus how well they do clinically.

Change management is a whole degree subject in itself, but to summarize, it involves changing opinions, challenging the status quo, education and being aware of any barriers to the new way of working – and having a strategy to deal with this.

You need to be passionate about what you are trying to do, but also approachable and adaptable; most of all, you need perseverance. Do not worry if you do not convince everyone to change practice straight away. You will get innovators and early adopters, and then late adopters. Social pressure will encourage the 'laggards' to change the way they work – as long as what you are proposing is in the patient's best interest and economically justifiable.

The key is allowing treatments to be implemented easily and having a system to ensure that this happens to every patient. An example of how you can ensure that treatment is underpinned by best available evidence is by using checklists or prompt cards to assist clinicians. This is something the authors of this textbook have experience doing within their own department. See http://chfg.org/guidance-documents/emergency-prompt-cards/.

An example of a prompt card is shown in Figure 15.1 for the treatment of a pulmonary embolus. The best available evidence shows that in specific situations, thrombolysis should be given. This card is explicit in how the treatment should be given and is an aide-memoire for how to implement the best available evidence from research papers to the patient, even in the heat of the moment.

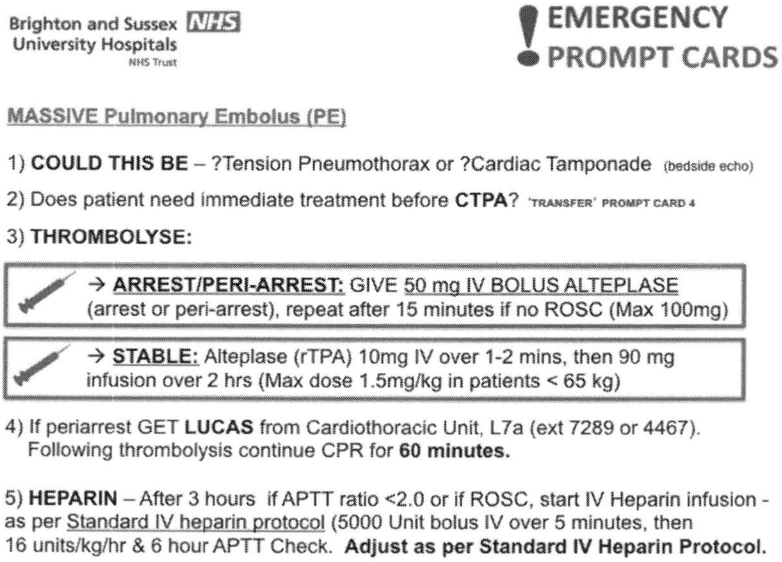

FIGURE 15.1 Example of a prompt card for treatment of pulmonary embolism using best available evidence.

A lot of this work has already been done so you can think about using nationally developed prompt cards as well as developing your own. Our and others' experience shows that these prompts can be helpful. They will help you take the evidence you read to the patients you treat. And that is essentially why we bother to read papers – *critical appraisal, from papers to patients.*

EVALUATING OUR PRACTICE AGAINST SET STANDARDS (THE AUDIT CYCLE)

Clinical audit is a process that aims to improve the quality of care or outcomes for patients using structured review of our clinical practice. It does not look to create new knowledge but rather seeks to ensure that existing knowledge is being used appropriately in departmental practice. The process is a circular one with audit leading to introduction of change, which then leads to re-audit. This is shown in Figure 15.2.

Preparing for an Audit

To audit you need an agreed evidence-based set of standards to compare your practice to. You can find these standards in many different ways:

- National quality indicators
- Nationally agreed guidelines – for example, the National Institute for Health and Care Excellence (NICE) or professional body guidelines
- Evidence from the literature – particularly from systematic reviews

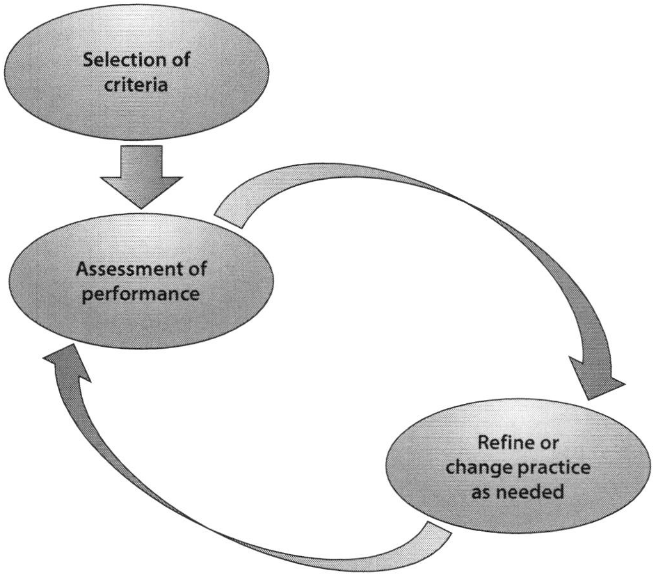

FIGURE 15.2 Clinical audit cycle.

- Current accepted local policies or protocols
- Local consensus opinion

These audit criteria should be SMART – specific, measurable, achievable and relevant, and there should be an appropriate timescale in which to do the audit.

Once the specifics of these standards are agreed, we can develop an audit protocol to compare them with our current practice. We can audit any aspect of patient care – how it is delivered, the processes involved or the outcomes.

Once the standard is agreed, the audit team must agree how many cases they should audit and the format of the audit. Generally, a selection of cases is all that is necessary. This sample should be big enough to ensure that the audit will fairly reflect current local practice but not so large that it becomes too onerous and therefore does not get completed. It is usual to pick the patients who form part of your audit in a consecutive fashion although a random selection or *n*th case may also be used. In addition, a decision whether the audit should be prospective or retrospective should be made prior to beginning the audit.

Performing an Audit

Once the structure of the audit has been decided, then the hard work of the audit begins. Patient notes need to be gathered, reviewed and the audit information gleaned from them. National audit studies recommend that at least 40 sets of notes should be reviewed. The size of the audit team depends on the number of notes to be reviewed. Generally, the data collected is kept in a database allowing for easy assessment of the information.

The results from the audit are compared to the agreed standards set out at the beginning of the audit. If your results are below the audit standard, then you should look at possible reasons for this. Ideally, you should critically assess why you are below the standard and make suggestions for steps you can put in place to help you improve. Once you have introduced these steps, you can re-audit to know whether there has been change. If your results are at or above the audit standard, then it is important for you not to sit on our laurels but to plan for a further audit in the future and see how you can improve care further. Remember that your audit might possibly be the victim of the Hawthorne effect (see the 'Glossary' at the end of the book).

It is important to present the audit in clinical governance meetings and suggest ways of making improvements. These suggestions must be a clear and specific action plan to follow, such as improved education or a new system of documentation.

When you make a change, be prepared to be in for the long haul and for any successes you have to drop off with time. This is the reason why re-audit is important.

MOVING BEYOND THE EVIDENCE BASE (RESEARCH)

Throughout this book we have been talking about critical appraisal. However, sometimes there is no evidence to base your decisions about your clinical practice on.

When there is no published evidence on which to base our decisions, we need to investigate – that is, perform research. Books have been written on how to perform research, and that is not the aim of this chapter. This section is just to highlight the stages involved in creating research.

The first step to creating research in any form is to come up with an appropriate clinical question. The clearer your clinical question, the easier it is to write your protocol and the more powerful your study will be.

High-level research is expensive, and therefore applying for funding is extremely important. There are many methods for obtaining this funding, and it is often dependent on the topic and type of research that you are going to perform.

On the basis of your clinical question you need to produce a protocol for your study and write a submission for ethical approval to the local ethics committee. Depending on the format and topic of your research, you may need to apply for regulatory approval as well.

To avoid publication bias, the study protocol should be made publically available, with a plan to publish the results regardless of what is found. An example of a repository for these trials can be found on websites such as https://clinicaltrials.gov.

Once all these steps have been completed you can begin to run your study and enrol patients. Once you have enrolled a sufficient quantity of patients, you can analyze the data that you have gathered and come to a conclusion. The whole research process can then be distilled into a clinical paper and published so that your experiences can be spread to the wider health care fraternity. See Figure 15.3.

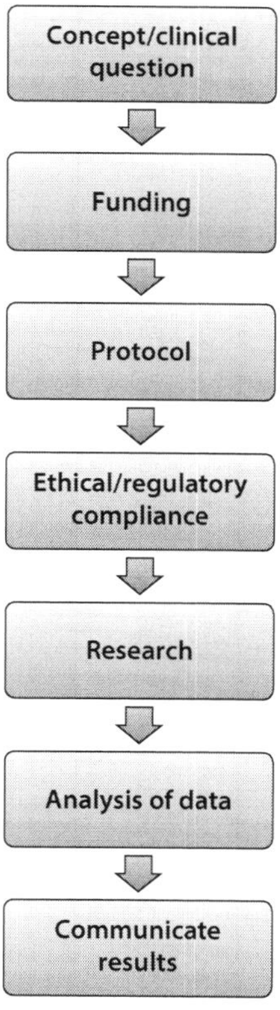

FIGURE 15.3 Steps to perform research.

Take-Home Message

1. Applying the known evidence to clinical care is imperative for good patient outcomes.
2. Clinical audit is used to assess your clinical practice; you are comparing your practice to an accepted set of clinical standards.
3. In research we seek new knowledge that will help us confirm or change our practice.

Section 5

Critical Appraisal Exams

16 An Approach to Critical Appraisal Exams

Let's face it – you may have bought this book to help you pass a critical appraisal exam. Critical appraisal is examined in all medical and allied health professions and at all levels. Learning how to appraise papers is an essential requirement for a health care professional – both to shape your practice as a 'best' evidence-based clinician and to help make decisions on departmental policies. So, it is understandable why critical appraisal is so frequently assessed. It is also understandable why people fear these exams so much, as critical appraisal can seem detached from the clinical work we are used to doing.

Exams can take the form of vivas, multiple choice questions and short answer questions. But the best way to assess someone's understanding of critical appraisal is an assessment of reading and understanding a paper you are given during an exam. It is this last type of assessment that the rest of this chapter concentrates on.

Most exams test your ability to critically appraise a paper and understand the process. It is not about turning you into a medical statistician. Whatever the specific exam, the questions are generally predictable and relevant, and require knowledge and understanding rather than rote formula learning; core concepts are most often examined and not 'far-out' minutiae.

But most importantly, most exams test what you need to know – that is, how will you assess the papers you read and how will that change your practice and departmental policy?

So why do people fail critical appraisal exams? There are generally three reasons: lack of preparation leading to lack of knowledge and understanding, lack of exam technique and lack of exam practice. By this point in the book, we have addressed the knowledge and understanding aspects, and over the next two chapters we move on to exam technique and practice.

Those candidates who have practiced with multiple mock exams often do the best. There are lots of mock exams out there – practice them in exam conditions with colleagues and discuss the answers together. Even better, find recent relevant papers, set your own exams and go over the answers. By practicing multiple papers, you will embed your skills and knowledge to make sure you pass. We have provided some mock examinations for you to use at the end of this section.

EXAM TECHNIQUE

Everybody who goes on an exam course or reads an exam preparation book thinks the exam technique section will just be common sense. There is no exception here, but (and a big but) there are specific tactics we would advise for critical appraisal exams.

The first thing to remember is that the exam is often very tight for time – especially if there is a long journal article. You must use your time very carefully. The key is reading the questions first and *then* reading the paper so you know where to concentrate your efforts. While reading the journal article, use a highlighter to make a note of key points, and write over the paper which question the key point is relevant to. Depending on the exam, the questions are usually predictable and may follow a standard format.

The best way to pass is make sure you get the full marks for the questions that require the least amount of effort. These are often questions which ask you to summarize the paper and if you would implement the finding. It goes without saying that you should write in a sensible and readable size – sadly, people have actually failed because of their handwriting. The examiners have multiple papers to mark, and so you need to make it easy for them to give you the marks. Write clearly and legibly. Writing in bullet points and underlining key points is acceptable, as is writing in capital letters.

Prior to answering any of the questions, there is one thing you must do. *It is imperative that you work out very quickly what type of paper you are reading.*

It should be very obvious what type of paper it is, but a large number of people who fail critical appraisal exams do so because they do not recognize what type of paper they are reading and thus how they should answer the questions. So, right at the start, think, is there a test being investigated (diagnostic paper), or is the paper looking at differences between two treatments (therapeutic paper)? Or is this an observational study?

The format of the questions changes across different types of exams, but there are usually the following types of questions:

- Writing a summary of the paper
- Questions about the design and methodology of the trial
- Questions about the statistics and results section, which may be simple calculations, for example, working out sensitivity and specificity
- Your interpretation of the strength and limitations of the paper and whether you would implement the results of the study

WRITING A SUMMARY

If your exam asks this, you are lucky as these are the easiest marks in the paper to get – so make sure you get them. The question will read something like this:

> Provide a 200-word or less summary of this paper in the box provided. Only the first 200 words will be considered – short bullet points are acceptable.

Do as the instructions say. Provide a summary – not your interpretation, not the whole paper regurgitated, not if you would implement their findings. Nothing but the summary – a bit like an informal version of what you would expect in the abstract.

The beauty of this question is that there are marks for literally copying sentences from the paper.

In many ways this is a brilliant but simple question – it asks if you have understood the paper well enough that you can distil it down to the abstract. You should have no problem with this as long as you have practiced doing this a number of times before the exam. When writing the summary, think about the following points:

- It needs to stand alone, so do not refer to other specific papers.
- There is no need to detail the background information.
- You need to include results as well as statistics (do not just say that the treatment worked or the test was good). You must include the primary outcome, but may wish to include some of the secondary outcomes if they were important.
- Use the author's conclusions, not your own.
- Do not write your opinion of the paper unless asked for it.
- *Beware that being asked to write a summary is not the same as being asked to write a checklist appraising the paper.*

What goes into a summary depends on the type of paper. Below, we have listed what should go into summaries of diagnostic, therapeutic and meta-nalysis papers, but of course with different types of papers different things needed to be mentioned in a summary.

It is often best if you start by writing out the headings and underlining them and then filling in the details as you go along. This makes it easier for the examiner to see where you have scored points. Bullet points are usually acceptable. The key sections are in italics:

Therapeutic Papers

Objectives
Design
Setting
Population
Methods
Intervention/treatment
Control
Outcome measurements
Results – State the results that the authors give, but it is especially important to give relative risk, number needed to treat and associated statistics as given in the paper
Conclusions

As with every list in medicine, there are various mnemonics to remember this by. We advise you to make up your own.

The key is to state that it is a therapeutic trial and how it was designed. You also must be sure to state the intervention and control. However, it can be hard to work out how much detail to put into this answer. An example is given here.

Austin et al. Effect of High-Flow Oxygen on Mortality in Chronic Obstructive Pulmonary Disease Patients in Pre-Hospital Setting: Randomized Controlled Trial. *BMJ* 2010;341:c5462

Question 1:

Provide a 200-word or less summary of this paper in the box provided. Only the first 200 words will be considered – short bullet points are acceptable.

Objective	To compare pre-hospital high-flow oxygen with titrated oxygen therapy for patients with acute exacerbations of chronic obstructive pulmonary disease.
Design	A therapeutic trial – interventional, non-blinded, cluster randomized, controlled, parallel group trial.
Setting	Pre-hospital patients attended by the Tasmanian Hospital Service between July 2006 and July 2007. All patients were admitted to the Royal Hobart Hospital, Tasmania.
Population	405 patients aged ≥35 years with breathlessness and a history or risk of chronic obstructive pulmonary disease (COPD). Risk of COPD defined as greater than 10-pack years.
Intervention and control	Titrated oxygen in the pre-hospital setting. High-flow oxygen in the pre-hospital setting.
Primary outcome	Pre-hospital and in-hospital mortality.
Results	An intention-to-treat analysis was performed. The mortality in the intervention group was 4% compared with 9% in the control group, and this reduction was significant (RR 0.42, 95 CI 0.20–0.89, p = 0.02). This was also true in those with confirmed COPD (RR0.22, 95% CI 0.05–0.91, p = 0.04). Titrated oxygen reduced therisk of death by 58% for all patients and 78% for those with COPD.
Conclusions	Compared with high-flow oxygen therapy, pre-hospital titrated oxygen therapy significantly reduced mortality in patients with acute exacerbations of COPD.

Diagnostic Papers

Objective
Design
Setting
Population
Methods
Test under investigation
Gold standard (good idea to mention if the test was done to all patients and if it was done blindly)
Results (positive predictive value, negative predictive value, sensitivity, specificity, likelihood ratio, Kappa); also quote the relevant statistics
Conclusion

Again, make sure you state that it is a diagnostic study and what is the test under investigation and the gold standard. Remember, they may not be as simple as an assay/radiological diagnosis. For example, in a test for appendicitis the gold standard could be operative findings plus follow-up for those who got discharged with a diagnosis of no appendicitis. In a similar way, the test may not be so easy to spot as a simple assay – it could be a clinical score, a set of rules or a combination of test and clinical score.

An example of a diagnostic summary is given here.

Diagnosis of Intussusception by Physician Novice Sonographers in the Emergency Department. Riera et al. *Ann Emerg Med.* 2012 September; 60(3):264–268.

Question 1:

Provide a 200-word or less summary of this paper in the box provided. Only the first 200 words will be considered – short bullet points are acceptable.

Objective	To investigate the performance characteristics of bedside ultrasound by paediatric emergency physicians who received limited and focused training in the diagnosis of ileocolic intussusception in children.
Design	Prospective diagnostic study.
Setting	Tertiary care children's hospital emergency department.
Population	Children with suspected ileocolic intussusception who were to undergo ultrasonography in the diagnostic radiology department.
Methods	Patients underwent bedside ultrasound performed by one of six emergency physicians attending or fellows who had received a 1-hour focused training session.
Test under investigation	Bedside ultrasound by an emergency physician.
Gold standard	Radiological department ultrasound.
Results	Bedside ultrasound had a sensitivity of 85% (95% CI54–97%), specificity of 97% (95% CI 89–99%), positive predictive value of 85% (95% CI 54–97%), negative predictive value of 97% (95% CI 89–99%), positive likelihood ratio of 29 (95% CI7.3–11.7) and negative likelihood ratio of 0.16 (95% CI 0.04–0.57).
Conclusion	This prospective observational study demonstrated the good performance characteristics of paediatric emergency physician-performed bedside ultrasonography for the diagnosis of intussusception in children after a single, focused training session.

Meta-Analysis

You should include the same headings as in the summary for the individual paper, but be sure to mention some specific extra points as shown below.

Paper identification
Paper selection
Funnel plot to see missing papers
Forest plot
Statistical analysis (including test for heterogeneity)

QUESTIONS ABOUT DESIGN AND METHODOLOGY

Knowledge and understanding are needed for this section. There may be questions directly related to the paper and there may be free-standing questions; for example, 'explain the importance of randomization'.

Again, technique is required. The length of your answer should be proportional to the marks allocated. There are some specific ways of answering the questions to help maximize marks.

1. Read the question. If it asks for a specific number of points, give that specific number of points. But if it says list the aspects of the design that were well done, then list all the factors you can think of starting with the most relevant, as long as it fits within the box.
2. If it asks for strength of the design, do not write strengths of the paper in general, but concentrate on the methodological design specifically. (See point 4 for further detail.)
3. You must explain 'buzz' words and not just put them in, in the hope that you will get some marks. For example, instead of stating that the study was pragmatic, state, 'The study was pragmatic in the fact that it was done with normal staff, using normal processes, with the type of patients we see and no special resources. Therefore the conclusions could easily be applied to our everyday practice'.
4. You must give attention to detail to your answers. For example, do not state that there was no loss to follow-up as an example of the strength of the design. This is careless as it is a *consequence* of the strength of the design. Instead you can say, 'The design of the study was excellent in that all patients would have a telephone follow-up and if they did not answer the phone, a home visit was arranged. This ensured that there was minimal loss to follow-up'.

The key, though, is to remember that different types of papers will have different things to look for when you are asked to assess the strengths of the design. Always think about design in terms of internal and external validity. Use the checklists that we have provided at the end of each chapter to help you assess the quality of the methodology.

QUESTIONS ABOUT RESULTS, STATISTICS AND 2 × 2 TABLES

These are easy marks to get if you have a good understanding of critical appraisal. You will not be expected to calculate p-values or power calculations, but in many exams you will be expected to understand how they are derived. You may be asked to calculate simple things based on the 2 × 2 tables, which are the key to the results section of many types of papers. For questions based on 2 × 2 tables, you will get the marks if you understand what you are calculating and can do it however the table is presented. You should start by stating the definitions and then always show your work for your calculations.

Two things that will help you score well in these questions are:

1. Know your definitions, for example, number needed to treat and sensitivity.
2. Be able to draw a standard 2 × 2 table no matter how the data is presented in the question or paper.

QUESTION ABOUT YOUR INTERPRETATION OF THE PAPER OR LIMITATIONS OF THE PAPER

These should be 'easy-ish' marks to get. There is often no definitive right or wrong answer, and marks can be awarded for coherent answers, whatever your interpretation of the paper.

The question will be put into a context of how they want you to answer it. For example, instead of saying, 'Is this paper any good?' the question will be something like 'Your new primary care lead heard about this paper and has asked if your general practice will be introducing the intervention. Explain what you would do if you were clinical lead and give your reasons'.

The best way to approach this question is to split your answer to cover different areas where marks can be gained:

1. What are the results? Are the differences in outcome significant or due to chance? Do not get confused by the difference between statistical significance ($p < 0.05$) and clinical significance (will it affect my patients?).
2. Is the methodology good enough for you to believe the results and conclusion – internal validity.
3. Decide if it could be generalized to your patients – external validity.
4. Decide if it is important for your patients. How common is the condition? What is the clinical significance of the result?
5. What could prevent implementation of the intervention in your place of work, and how easy would the identified barriers be to overcome? Think about the four barriers to implementation – they all begin with B:
   a. Badness: What harm could be caused by the intervention?
   b. Burden of disease: Is it so rare that no one cares?
   c. Budget: Can we afford to make the changes?
   d. Beliefs: How will we educate people about this new intervention, and how will we deal with intransigent colleagues?

Take-Home Message

1. At the beginning work out what type of study it is.
2. Read the questions before you read the paper.
3. Answer the easy questions first – first and last questions.
4. When considering your opinion of the paper, consider internal and external validity.

---

17 Practice Papers

Please note that both practice papers are fictitious. Do not go implementing what is in these papers!

PRACTICE PAPER 1

ρ-BRB as a Diagnostic Marker of Bacterial Infection in the Emergency Department

Coughlan EP, Galloway RI, Bootland DJ
Department of Emergency Medicine, Brighton

Introduction

Sepsis is a significant cause of death, causing 37,000 deaths in the United Kingdom annually.[1] The Surviving Sepsis Guidelines 2012 recommend early recognition, resuscitation and administration of antibiotics.[2] Early recognition and intervention saves lives. However, some patients with an infection have minimal or even no symptoms or signs, making early recognition difficult.[3]

Diagnostic tests such as white cell count (WCC), C-reactive protein (CRP) and procalcitonin have all been used to try to identify septic patients early and provide information on prognosis.[4–6]

Serum ρ-BRB (rho-B-cell reticular bioprotein) is a 225–amino acid peptide, produced by B-cells on release of antibodies. The rho isomer of the B-cell reticular protein is produced when antibodies are produced against bacterial infection. The level of this in the bloodstream should correspond to the degree of the body's response and hence to the severity of the infection. The presence of high levels of this protein in the bloodstream should indicate a need for antibiotics.

We assessed the diagnostic ability of serum ρ-BRB to diagnose an infection (as determined by positive sputum or blood cultures). We hypothesized that for patients who present to the emergency department (ED), ρ-BRB would be more sensitive than CRP and WCC as a marker of the presence of bacterial infection.

Methods

The study was performed between March and September 2013 in the ED of a tertiary referral hospital with 150,000 attendances per year. This was a prospective study of patients presenting to a tertiary university hospital. Consecutive adult patients (aged over 18 years) who presented to our ED with signs and symptoms suggestive of a respiratory tract infection and who required phlebotomy were enrolled into the study after consent was obtained by one of the study personnel. Signs and symptoms of infection included cough, wheeze, productive sputum, shortness of breath, pyrexia and chest pain. Patients were excluded if they had a recently diagnosed infection, if they were already on antibiotics or if they had a recognized cause of reduced immunity (e.g. autoimmune disease, diabetes, taking chemotherapeutic agents and taking steroids).

Baseline characteristics were obtained for all patients enrolled. Blood was also taken so that it could be tested for full blood count, C-reactive protein and serum ρ-BRB. Samples of blood and sputum were taken for culture. Staff responsible for processing of cultures and blood tests did so independently without knowledge of the results of other samples. Treating clinicians were kept unaware of the results of the serum ρ-BRB throughout the study. The study was approved by the hospital ethics committee and verbal consent was obtained from patients for the additional sampling.

Data Analysis

The best cutoff value was chosen using Youden's index. During statistical analysis the Mann–Whitney U-test was used to compare independent samples and the chi-squared test was used to compare proportions. All tests were two-sided and a p-value of 0.05 was considered significant. Statistical analysis was performed using StatsforU (Rahaman Software, Brighton, United Kingdom).

Results

Over the 6-month period, 700 patients were enrolled into the study. Patients ranged in age from 19 to 103 years of age with a mean of 64 years and a median age of 65 years. Sixty percent of patients were male. Twenty-seven percent of patients in total had a positive culture (either sputum or blood). See Table 17.1.

To assess the ρ-BRB test, we drew a receiver operating characteristic (ROC) curve (see Figure 17.1). Cutoff values were used every 20 ng/L from 20 to 160 ng/L (see Table 17.2), and the sensitivity and specificity of the test were assessed at each of these levels.

Figure 17.1 shows a ROC curve illustrating the sensitivity and (1-specificity) of ρ-BRB. The area under the ROC curve was 0.93. After assessing each of the cutoff values, the optimum level for the ρ-BRB test was found to be 40 ng/L.

TABLE 17.1
Baseline Characteristics of Patients in Respect to Culture Results

	Positive Cultures (95% CI), n = 189	Negative Cultures (95% CI), n = 511
Age (years)	76.6 (74.0–79.2)	59.8 (57.4–62.2)
Sex (M:F)	115:74	304:207
WCC (/mm3)	11.6 (9.7–13.6)	10.2 (8.3–12.2)
CRP	56.3 (47.2–65.4)	14.8 (11.7–17.8)
ρ-BRB	124 (114.5–133.5)	30.4 (26.1–34.6)

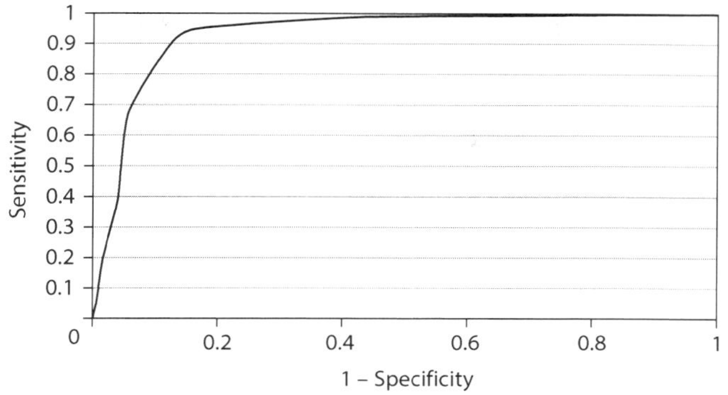

FIGURE 17.1 ROC curve for ρ-BRB.

TABLE 17.2
Sensitivity and Specificity for Different Cutoff Values for ρ-BRB

Cutoff Levels (ng/L)	Sensitivity	Specificity
20	0.99	0.60
40	0.94	0.85
60	0.84	0.90
80	0.70	0.94
100	0.61	0.95
120	0.44	0.96
140	0.32	0.97
160	0.27	0.97

The threshold values of a white cell count greater than 12,000/mm^3 and less than 4000/mm^3 were chosen to mirror the diagnostic criteria of SIRS (Systemic inflammatory response syndrome) in an attempt to improve its sensitivity. At that value, in this study, white cell count had a sensitivity of 36% and a specificity of 30% for diagnosing the presence of bacterial infection.

The normal CRP value of <10 mg/L was chosen as this is the current accepted value from the literature. Using this cutoff, CRP had a sensitivity of 66% and a specificity of 84%.

From the ROC curve we calculated the optimum value for ρ-BRB to be 40 ng/L. At this cutoff level, of the 189 positive culture results, 178 people had a positive ρ-BRB (>40 ng/L). Of 511 patients in the negative culture group, 433 had a negative ρ-BRB (40 ng/L). This gives us a sensitivity of 94% and a specificity of 85% (Table 17.3).

Discussion

The diagnosis of bacterial infection even in the acutely unwell patient is extremely difficult. The balance between prescribing antibiotics for those with a bacterial

TABLE 17.3
Sensitivity and Specificity for White Cell Counts, C-Reactive Protein and ρ-BRB

	Sensitivity %	Specificity %
WCC (>12,000 or <4000/mm^3)	36 (68/189) (95% CI 30–42)	70 (358/511) (95% CI 64–76)
CRP (>10 mg/L)	66 (126/189) (95% CI 60–72)	84 (429/511) (95% CI 80–88)
ρ-BRB (> 40 ng/L)	94 (178/189) (95% CI 90–98)	85 (433/511) (95% CI 81–89)

infection, who if left untreated may develop sepsis, and not prescribing antibiotics for those who do not have a bacterial infection is a difficult one. There are significant potential risks for the individual patient and indeed to society if the wrong decision is made. The use of clinical history, examination and clinician gestalt has long been recognized as being insufficient if used in isolation.[3]

Many tests have been used to aid the identification of patients who required treatment with antibiotics. White cell counts are used daily in every hospital to aid in the diagnosis. In the meta-analysis by Wallman et al., white cell count was found to have a low sensitivity (36%) but to improve the specificity (81%) of clinical examination and clinician gestalt.[4] These findings have been mirrored in this study.

C-reactive protein was initially discovered in 1930. It is a non-specific marker of inflammation, which rises in the presence of bacterial infection. It is often used in combination with clinical examination and clinician gestalt to diagnose bacterial infection. Although quite specific, it suffers from a lower sensitivity. The values we found (sensitivity of 66% and specificity of 84%) for CRP are similar to those of other studies.

ρ-BRB is a new test for the diagnosis of bacterial infection. In this study we found it to have a sensitivity of 94% (95% confidence interval [CI] 90–98) and a specificity of 85% (95% CI 81–89) when the cutoff value of 40 ng/L is used. The high sensitivity of this test compared with other markers of bacterial infection makes it extremely helpful in ruling out the need for antibiotics with a serum ρ-BRB of less than 40.

Further studies should focus on the use of this test in conjunction with other tests, such as procalcitonin, to hopefully improve the sensitivity so that the combination can be used as a rule-out test.

Conclusions

The high sensitivity of this test may potentially allow us to rule out bacterial infection in patients and reduce the inappropriate prescription of antibiotics.

Competing Interests

Dr Coughlan has received a bursary from Apex Pharmaceuticals to present this work at the ACEP conference in California.

REFERENCES

1. O'Riordan S, Finn M. The epidemiology of sepsis. *BJM* 2009, 21(3): 431–435.
2. Surviving sepsis campaign: International guidelines for management of severe sepsis and septic shock. *Critical Care Medicine* 2013, 41(2): 580–637.
3. Ransom P, McKenzie M, Duff M. Sepsis presentations to a tertiary referral center: Clinician gestalt is not enough. *JoS* 2010, 15(4): 2130–2138.
4. Wallman P, Beadsworth A, Bryant G. The use of white cell count as a prognostic indicator of infection: A meta-analysis. *JoS* 2008, 13(6): 2860–2873.
5. Nelson M, Cottingham R. C-reactive protein in bacterial infection, a review of the current literature. *JoS* 2011, 16(1): 540–561.
6. Ghani R, Rahaman A. Procalcitonin as a marker of significant bacterial infection presenting to the emergency department. *JoS* 2012, 17(6): 3142–3161.

PRACTICE PAPER 1: QUESTIONS

Bootland et al. ρ-BRB as a Diagnostic Marker of Bacterial Infection in the Emergency Department

Question 1

Provide a 200-word or less summary of this paper in the box provided. Only the first 200 words will be considered – short bullet points are acceptable. (Maximum of 7 marks)

Question 2

1. Describe your understanding of a confidence interval. (2 marks)
2. Is this more or less useful than a p-value? (2 marks)
3. The mean (95% CI) for age in the positive culture group was 76.6 (74.0–79.2) and in the negative culture group was 59.8 (57.4–62.2). If the CIs do not meet, what does this mean? (2 marks)

Question 3

Give three aspects of the methodology of this study that you consider were good. (3 marks)

Question 4

What is meant by the reference (gold) standard test? What do you think of the gold standard test in this study? (2 marks)

Question 5

What do you understand as sensitivity and specificity? What is meant by the area under the curve in respect to ROC curves? (2 marks)

Question 6

From the statement 'Of the 189 positive culture results, 178 people had a positive ρ-BRB (> 40 ng/L); of 511 patients in the negative culture group, 433 had a negative ρ-BRB (40 ng/L)' draw a 2 × 2 table and showing all your workings. Calculate the following (8 marks):

1. Sensitivity
2. Specificity
3. Positive predictive value
4. Negative predictive value
5. Positive likelihood ratio
6. Negative likelihood ratio

Question 7

Your chief executive read this paper. He feels that we should get this test into the laboratory and that it will save the trust money by reducing the prescription of antibiotics. What will you say to him? (4 marks)

PRACTICE PAPER 1: ANSWERS

Bootland et al. ρ-BRB as a Diagnostic Marker of Bacterial Infection in the Emergency Department

Question 1

Provide a 200-word or less summary of this paper in the box provided. Only the first 200 words will be considered – short bullet points are acceptable. (Maximum of 7 marks)

Objectives: To assess the diagnostic capability of serum ρ-BRB in making a diagnosis of bacterial infection and to compare it with WCC and CRP.

Design: Diagnostic observation study.

Setting: Emergency department of a tertiary referral hospital with 150,000 attendances per year.

Population: Consecutive adults over 18 with signs and symptoms suggestive of a respiratory tract infection and who required phlebotomy. Patients were excluded if they had a recently diagnosed infection, were already on treatment or had a recognized cause of reduced immunity.

Test under investigation: ρ-BRB.

Gold standard: Positive culture of blood or sputum.

Results: A ROC curve was performed for ρ-BRB with the area under the curve of 0.93 and optimal cutoff value of 40 ng/L. At this cutoff level ρ-BRB had a sensitivity of 94% (90–98 95% CI) and a specificity of 85% (81–89 95% CI). The sensitivity of ρ-BRB was better than those of both WCC (36%) and CRP (66%).

Conclusions: The high sensitivity of this test may potentially allow us to rule out bacterial infection in patients and reduce the inappropriate prescription of antibiotics.

180 words

Question 2

1. Describe your understanding of a confidence interval. (2 marks)
2. Is this more or less useful than a p-value? (2 marks)
3. The mean (95% CI) for age in the positive culture group was 76.6 (74.0–79.2) and in the negative culture group was 59.8 (57.4–62.2). If the CIs do not meet, what does this mean? (2 marks)

1. Confidence intervals: This is a range in which the population value is likely to lie.
2. p-Values give you a yes or no answer to whether a result is statistically significant or not, whereas a CI gives you a range in which the population value is likely to lie. Confidence intervals are generally considered to be more clinically valuable as they allow you to interpret the likely size of the effect.
3. It means that there is a statistically significant difference between the two groups in respect to age because the CIs do not overlap.

Question 3

Give three aspects of the methodology of this study that you consider were good. (3 marks)

(In the exam, you would only need to give three points – but we have listed all possibilities.)

- It is a prospective study, which is generally regarded as higher quality than retrospective studies.
- Consecutive patients were enrolled reducing the chance for selection bias, that is, reducing the chance that researchers influence which patients get enrolled. This form of sampling is more likely than convenience sampling to be representative of your population.
- The inclusion and exclusion criteria are pragmatic and yet excluded important subgroups that might have influenced the test.
- All patients had the gold standard test and the test under investigation and they were assessed independently of each other.
- A ROC curve was drawn to assess the most appropriate cutoff value for the test.

Question 4

What is meant by the reference (gold) standard test? What do you think of the gold standard test in this study? (2 marks)

> The gold standard test is the best test available to diagnose a condition, it should be used as the comparison test in diagnostic studies looking at the ability of a novel test to detect the same disease.
>
> The gold standard test was a culture sample and was inappropriate in this study. The absence of a positive culture does not exclude bacterial infection. As such many of the patients who have a negative culture may have had a bacterial cause for their symptoms.
>
> A better gold standard would be discharge diagnosis (which would be based on clinical examination and history, imaging, relevant blood and pathology tests and a period of observation).

Question 5

What do you understand as sensitivity and specificity? What is meant by the area under the curve in respect to ROC curves? (2 marks)

> **Sensitivity:** The proportion of people with the disease who test positive. It is useful for those who are interested in 'how good is this test', for example, clinical biochemists. A high sensitivity tells us a test is good at ruling out disease in a patient who tests negative (SnOut).
>
> **Specificity:** The proportion of people without the disease who test negative. It is useful for those who are interested in 'how good is this test', for example, clinical biochemists. A high specificity tells us a test is good at ruling in a disease in a patient who tests positive (SpIn).
>
> The area under the ROC curve is a measure of how accurate a test is. It is measured between 0 and 1; the closer to 1, the better the test.

Question 6

From the statement 'Of the 189 positive culture results, 178 people had a positive ρ-BRB (> 40 ng/L); of 511 patients in the negative culture group, 433 had a negative ρ-BRB (40 ng/L)' draw a 2×2 table and showing all your workings. Calculate the following (8 marks):

1. Sensitivity
2. Specificity
3. Positive predictive value
4. Negative predictive value
5. Positive likelihood ratio
6. Negative likelihood ratio

		Gold Standard	
		Culture Positive	Culture Negative
Test under	>40 ng/L	178 (a)	78 (b)
Investigation	<40 ng/L	11 (c)	433 (d)

1. Sensitivity: Proportion of people with the disease who test positive
   = a/a + c
   = 178/(178 + 11) = 178/189 = 0.94
2. Specificity: Proportion of people without the disease who test negative
   = d/(b + d)
   = 433/(78 + 433) = 433/511 = 0.85
3. PPV: Proportion of people with a positive test who have the disease
   = a/(a + b)
   = 178/(178 + 78) = 178/256 = 0.70
4. NPV: Proportion of people with a negative test who do not have the disease
   = d/(c + d)
   = 433/(11 + 433) = 433/444 = 0.98
5. Positive likelihood ratio
   = How much more likely is a positive test to be found in a person with the disease (sensitivity) compared with/without the disease (False positive = 1 – Specificity)
   = Sensitivity/1 – Specificity
   = 0.94/(1 – 0.85) = 0.94/0.15 = 6.3
   (or from first principles = [a/(a + c)]/[b/(b + d)]
6. Negative likelihood ratio
   = How much more likely is a –ve test in a person with the disease (False negative = 1 –Sensitivity) compared with a –ve test without the disease (specificity)
   = (1– Sensitivity)/Specificity
   = (1 – 0.94)/0.85 = 0.06/0.85 = 0.07
   (or from first principles = [c/(c + a)]/[d/(d + b)]

In the actual exam you will get mathematics, which are numerically easier to do – you would never fail for a lack of multiple division knowledge.

Question 7

Your chief executive read this paper. He feels that we should get this test into the laboratory and that it will save the trust money by reducing the prescription of antibiotics. What will you say to him? (4 marks)

Politely decline this suggestion on the basis of:

- It is a single-centre study and as such external validity is not assured.
- Although the gold standard used should diagnose a positive infection in patients, there will be a large percentage of the patients with a negative culture who also had a bacterial infection and as such should have antibiotics to prevent worsening of their illness; that is, the internal validity is not good as the gold standard used in this paper is not appropriate.
- The sensitivity is too low to use it as a rule-out test; hence you could not safely choose not to give antibiotics to these patients (poor applicability).
- No cost analysis was performed and as such we cannot know the cost of introducing the test, and the daily cost of doing the test would reduce antibiotic costs even if the test did have the sensitivity to rule out the need for antibiotics (poor applicability).

PRACTICE PAPER 2: JOURNAL ARTICLE

Provision of Tea and Coffee in the ED to Reduce 'Left without Being Seen' Rates

Coughlan EP, Galloway RI, Bootland DJ
Royal Sussex County Hospital, Brighton

Introduction

In 2011, in response to concerns over the utility of the 4-hour rule, the UK government introduced a new set of eight quality indicators (QIs) which it was claimed would act as a better measure of the care that National Health Service (NHS) emergency departments (EDs) provide. After further consultation, the QIs were altered such that EDs are now measured against five 'headline' QIs, and these are divided into two main groups: patient impact (unplanned re-attendance and left without being seen [LWBS]) and timeliness (time to initial assessment, time to treatment and total time in the ED). Performance is currently judged against each group rather than each QI although total time in the ED (essentially equivalent to the old 4-hour rule) remains as a stand-alone measure.

The measure of left without being seen 'reflects the satisfaction of patients with the initial management experience they receive'.[1] Leaving before being seen by a clinical decision maker also represents clinical risk, and it has been demonstrated that 49% of patients who are leaving before being seen subsequently require urgent treatment.[1] The QIs suggest departments should not have LWBS rates at or above 5%. In our region, LWBS rates are currently running at a level of 6%.[2]

Achievement of the standards against the QIs has proved challenging for many departments and has resulted in novel methods of improving quality. A recent telephone survey of patients from this department who had been designated as LWBS highlighted lack of comfort in the waiting area as a major cause of failure to wait to be seen.[3] We hypothesized that provision of free tea and coffee in the waiting room for both patients and relatives would reduce our LWBS rate and improve the service experience of patients attending the department.

Methods

Patients

The study population comprised all adult patients (age ≥ 18 years) presenting to one of four UK district general hospital (DGH) EDs in the south of England over 1 week in August 2012. Patients admitted directly to a 'resus' cubicle, whether having been transported to hospital by ambulance or arriving by private transport, were excluded from the study.

Randomization

Due to the nature of the study, cluster randomization was deemed the most appropriate means of randomization. We invited four DGHs to be involved in the study and used computer-generated random numbers to cluster randomize them to the intervention or control group. Neither the patients nor the treating ED team were blinded to the group that their hospital had been randomized to. The local ethics committee waived the need for patients' consent.

Intervention

EDs randomized to the intervention group were provided with an automated tea- and coffee-making machine that was to be placed within the main seating area of the ED waiting room. Complimentary contracts with the owners of the vending machines were negotiated for the duration of the trial to ensure daily maintenance and stocking checks for each hospital in the intervention group. EDs in the control group were to leave their waiting rooms standard – none of the hospitals in the control group routinely provided free drinks for people in their waiting rooms.

Data Collection

Patients' movement through the department or leaving before being seen was recorded as routinely done by each department. Demographic data, length of wait to be seen, pain score and final diagnosis on discharge from the ED were also recorded by each department's computerized patient system. On a weekly basis this data was retrospectively retrieved by four research nurses and entered into a computer database. A subset of the patients in each group was surveyed by a research nurse via telephone questionnaire to assess their satisfaction with their attendance in the ED. Patient satisfaction was measured using the Hartland questionnaire that has been validated in similar populations[4]; the Hartland score measures patient satisfaction on a scale of 0–10, with a change of 1 point considered to be significant.

Outcome Measures

The primary outcome measure was rate of patients who left without being seen by a clinical decision maker – defined as a post-registration doctor or emergency nurse practitioner (ENP). Secondary outcome measures were patient satisfaction and waiting time.

Statistical Analysis

Statistical analysis software that is routinely available commercially (SPSS™) was used to analyze the data. The primary outcome measure was reported as a proportion of the total number of attendances, and a test of independent proportions was performed with a chi-squared test. Secondary outcome measures were normally distributed and thus analyzed using Student's t-test.

Previous work by Parker et al.[5] demonstrated a 3% absolute difference in LWBS after an intervention to improve comfort in the ED waiting area. We calculated that a total of 2400 patients would be required to demonstrate a reduction from 7% in the control arm to 4% in the intervention arm, with a power of 0.80 and a type 1 error rate of 0.05.

Results

During the study period, 2527 patients attended the four EDs enrolled in the study. Of these, 91 patients were subsequently found to have incomplete data, predominantly due to having a discharge diagnosis and location recorded as 'unclassified'. As such 2436 patient attendances were analyzed: 1272 in the control group and 1164 in the intervention group (Figure 17.2).

Characteristics of the study groups are given in Table 17.4, and it can be seen that the two groups did not differ in terms of gender or age.

The rates of patients classified as LWBS are shown in Table 17.5

The overall LWBS rate was statistically different between the two groups (relative risk [RR] 0.63, 95% CI 0.45–0.90, $p = 0.04$) with a LWBS rate in the control group of 6.37% and in the intervention group 4.04%. This was particularly true in the patients classified as 'minors' (RR 0.42, 95% CI 0.27–0.66, $p < 0.001$).

The time that patients waited to be seen by a doctor or nurse practitioner was slightly longer in the control group (79 minutes, 95% CI 78.1–80.5) than in the intervention group (75 minutes, 95% CI 72.7–76.3), and although small, and thus unlikely to be of importance, this difference was statistically significant ($p < 0.001$) (Table 17.6).

Patient satisfaction scores were obtained from a randomly selected subgroup of 200 patients (100 patients in each group; 20 medical, 20 surgical and 60 minors). There was a statistically significant improvement in patient satisfaction for those allocated to the intervention arm of the study ($p = 0.007$), and again this was most marked in the patients classified as 'minors' (Table 17.7).

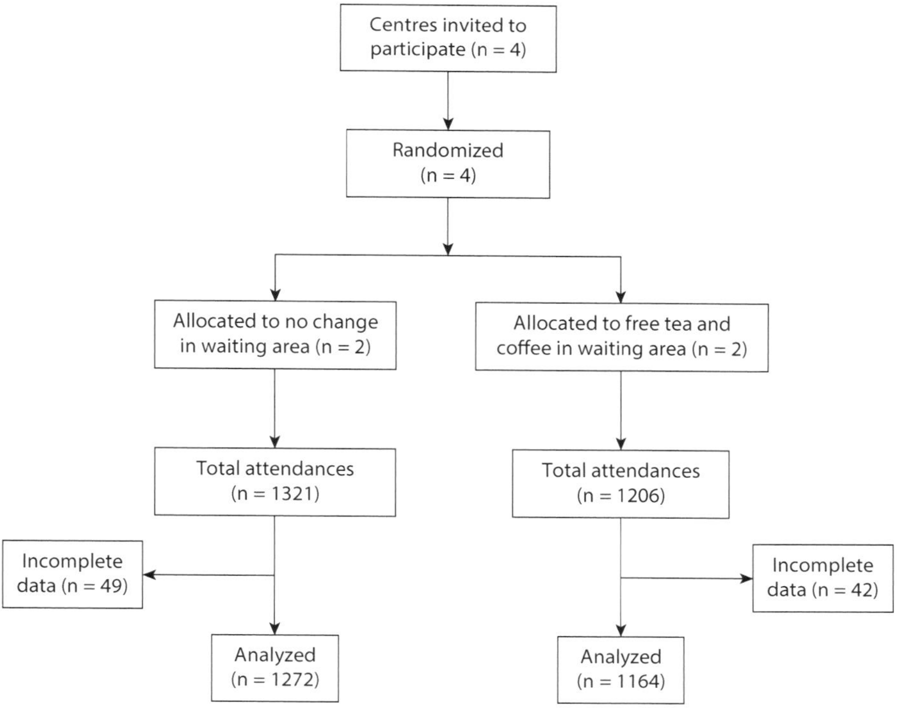

FIGURE 17.2 Patient flow diagram.

TABLE 17.4
Study Group Characteristics

Population Characteristics	Total Population	Interventional Group	Control Group	p-Value
		Sex, No. (%)		
Male	1368 (56)	660 (57)	708 (56)	
Female	1068 (44)	504 (43)	564 (44)	0.227
Age, years, mean (SD)	61.8 (1.4)	61.6 (1.3)	61.9 (1.4)	0.86
		Mode of Arrival, No. (%)		
Ambulance	504 (21)	192 (16)	312 (25)	<0.001
Private transport	1932 (79)	972 (84)	960 (75)	
		Diagnosis Group, No. (%)		
Medical	704 (29)	184 (16)	520 (41)	<0.001
Surgical	252 (10)	108 (9)	144 (11)	
Minor injury	1480 (61)	872 (75)	608 (48)	
		Admission Status, No. (%)		
Admitted	824 (34)	288 (25)	476 (37)	<0.001
Discharged	1612 (66)	876 (75)	796 (63)	

TABLE 17.5
Patients Classified as Left without Being Seen

	Total Population		Intervention Group		Control Group		
Diagnostic Group	Number	Percentage (95% CI)	Number	Percentage (95% CI)	Number	Percentage (95% CI)	p-Value
Medical	34	4.83	10	5.43	24	4.62	0.69
Surgical	17	6.75	8	7.41	9	6.25	0.80
Minors	77	5.20	29	3.33	48	7.89	<0.001
Overall	128	5.25	47	4.04	81	6.37	0.013

TABLE 17.6
Waiting Time to Be Seen by Decision Maker (Minutes)

	Total Population (Mean)	Intervention Group (Mean)	Control Group (Mean)	p-Value
Medical	83	93	79	<0.001
Surgical	89	97	83	<0.001
Minors	72	68	78	<0.001
Overall	77	75	79	<0.001

TABLE 17.7
Patient Satisfaction: Hartland Score

	Total Population (Mean)	Intervention Group (Mean)	Control Group (Mean)	p-Value
Medical	8.3	8.2	8.5	0.32
Surgical	8.1	7.9	8.2	0.39
Minors	8.1	8.5	7.6	<0.001
Overall	8.0	8.3	7.9	0.007

Discussion

Our study showed that implementation of access to free tea and coffee in the waiting areas of UK DGH EDs significantly reduced the rates of patients leaving before being seen from 6.4% to 4.0% in the two groups, a reduction that would see hospitals achieve the NHS target of a LWBS rate of less than 5%. Although the intervention had its largest effect in those classified as having 'minor injuries', it is important to note that the statistical significance of the result was maintained for all patients.

Although LWBS rates are perhaps intuitively clinically unimportant or certainly less important than clinical outcome measures such as pain scores and mortality, as has been highlighted by the UK government, they can be seen to be reliable surrogates for the standard of care that EDs provide. Nevertheless, it is reassuring to note that not only were LWBS rates reduced by the intervention we studied, but also patient satisfaction scores in the intervention group were statistically higher than those in the control group. This suggests that this intervention has the rare ability to please clinicians, administrators and patients.

We believe this is the first prospective randomized controlled study to look at the impact of changes to improve comfort in the ED waiting area. Parker et al.[5] previously performed a single-centre pilot study with a retrospective control group looking at more general improvements in factors associated with patient comfort in the waiting area and demonstrated a 3% absolute reduction in LWBS rates between their before and after groups. The problems of retrospective and single-centre studies are widely acknowledged, but it is interesting to note that we found a similar absolute reduction in LWBS rates after implementation of a measure to improve the patient and relative experience.

The trial has a few limitations that are worthy of discussion. The lack of sufficient funding did not enable us to capture patient satisfaction scores at the time of their visit, and thus these had to be done retrospectively by telephone. Equally, the size of the trial meant that it was not possible to follow up every patient, and thus we had to be satisfied only with a small sample of the population studied rather than the whole population, as would have been done in an ideal world. Finally, there is an inherent problem in offering food or drink to patients who may have needed surgical intervention early during their hospital visit. As such, it was left to the discretion of the individual ED to manage how best to advise this subset of patients attending the ED if free beverages were available. It was not possible either to identify these patients or to exclude them from the analysis, but we felt this was justified as part of the pragmatic study design.

Conclusion

This multicentre randomized controlled trial demonstrated a significant reduction in LWBS rates and improvements in patient satisfaction after implementation of free tea and coffee in the waiting area of UK EDs, particularly those classified as having 'minor injuries'. Such interventions are likely to improve not only the patient experience but also the ability of UK EDs to demonstrate their high standard of care through achievement of the LWBS QI and thus should be recommended to trusts.

REFERENCES

1. A&E Clinical Quality Indicators Implementation Guidance. Department of Health. Downloaded from http://www.dh.gov.uk/prod_consum_dh/groups/dh_digitalassets/@dh/@en/@ps/documents/digitalasset/dh_123055.pdf on May 3, 2012.
2. Galloway R, Coughlan E, Bootland D. An audit of left without being seen (LWBS) rates in six hospitals in the south of England. *J Crit Apprais* 2011;1:52–54.
3. Body D, Coughlan E. Telephone survey of those leaving the emergency department without being seen. *UK Med J* 2011;88:116–117.
4. Houghtan T, Smith J. The Hartland patient satisfaction scale – A validation study in a UK emergency department. *J Inv Med* 2006;26:14–18.
5. Parker S, Sadek S, O'Riordan S. Do improvements in comfort in the waiting area result in fewer patients leaving without being seen? A pilot study. *J Crit Apprais* 2011;2:102–105.

PRACTICE PAPER 2: QUESTIONS

Coughlan et al. Provision of Tea and Coffee in the ED to Reduce 'Left without Being Seen' Rates

QUESTION 1

Provide a 200-word or less summary of this paper in the box provided. Only the first 200 words will be considered – short bullet points are acceptable. (Maximum of 7 marks)

Question 2

1. What is cluster randomization? (1 mark)
2. Give one advantage and one disadvantage of cluster randomization. (2 marks)

Question 3

The following excerpt is taken from the text:

Previous work by Parker et al.[5] demonstrated a 3% absolute difference in LWBS after an intervention to improve comfort in the ED waiting area. We calculated that a total of 2400 patients would be required to demonstrate a reduction from 7% in the control arm to 4% in the intervention arm, with a power of 0.80 and a type 1 error rate of 0.05.

1. What is meant by the power of a study? (1 mark)
2. Do you think the power of this study was appropriate? (1 mark)
3. What is meant by type 1 and type 2 errors? Give an example of each. (2 marks)

Question 4

1. What is the difference between a primary and a secondary outcome measure? (1 mark)
2. What is the difference between qualitative and quantitative data? (1 mark)
3. In this study, are the secondary outcome measures quantitative or qualitative data? Explain your answer. (3 marks)

Question 5

1. What does a p-value represent? (2 marks)
2. What is meant by CONSORT statement? (2 marks)

Question 6

The following table was produced from a follow-up study in different hospitals but run with identical methodology. Calculate the absolute risk reduction (ARR), the relative risk, the relative risk reduction (RRD) and the number needed to treat (NNT). (5 marks)

	LWBS	Waited to Be Seen
Free Tea and Coffee	330	610
No Free Tea and Coffee	410	530

Question 7

Your chief executive has read this paper and tells you she wants you to use some of the ED budget to provide free tea and coffee in the waiting room. What will you say to her? (6 marks)

PRACTICE PAPER 2: ANSWERS

Coughlan et al. Provision of Tea and Coffee in the ED to Reduce 'Left without Being Seen' Rates

Question 1

Provide a 200-word or less summary of this paper in the box provided. Only the first 200 words will be considered – short bullet points are acceptable. (Maximum of 7 marks)

Objectives: To see if provision of free tea and coffee in the waiting room reduces LWBS rate and improves the service experience of patients attending the ED.
Design: A therapeutic, randomized controlled trial.
Setting: Four district general hospital EDs in the south of England during 1 week in August 2012.
Population: All adult (≥18 years) patients presenting to the ED; patients admitted to the resuscitation area were excluded.
Methods: Patients were randomized by cluster with receiving hospital being the unit of randomization. Neither patients nor treating clinicians were blinded to the interventions.
Intervention/treatment: Automated free tea and coffee machine available in the waiting room.
Control: Standard waiting room.
Outcome measures: Primary outcome measure was the rate of patients who left without having been seen by a clinical decision maker.
Results: The overall LWBS rate was statistically different between the two groups (RR 0.63, 95% CI 0.45–0.90, $p = 0.04$), with a LWBS rate in the control group of 6.37% and in the intervention group 4.04%.
Conclusions: This trial demonstrated a significant reduction in LWBS rates and improvements in patient satisfaction after implementation of free tea and coffee in the waiting area.

Question 2

1. What is cluster randomization? (1 mark)
2. Give one advantage and one disadvantage of cluster randomization. (2 marks)

1. Cluster randomization is when the unit of randomization is not an individual study participant but rather a group of individuals treated in the same place or by the same person.

2.

Advantages:

Cluster randomization allows us to study interventions which are applied to groups rather than individuals, such as process changes such as the introduction of a clinical decision unit (CDU). If we were to try having two different processes operating in the same clinical area (e.g. some patients having access to a CDU and others not), there is the potential for confusion, protocol violation and bias; cluster randomization works to avoid this.

Disadvantages:

Cluster randomization tends to require a greater complexity of design and analysis.

Question 3

The following excerpt is taken from the text:

> Previous work by Parker et al.[5] demonstrated a 3% absolute difference in LWBS after an intervention to improve comfort in the ED waiting area. We calculated that a total of 2400 patients would be required to demonstrate a reduction from 7% in the control arm to 4% in the intervention arm, with a power of 0.80 and a type 1 error rate of 0.05.

1. What is meant by the power of a study? (1 mark)
2. Do you think the power of this study was appropriate? (1 mark)
3. What is meant by type 1 and type 2 errors? Give an example of each. (2 marks)

1. In most studies we are interested in whether there is an association between two variables, for example does given drug X result in reduce mortality. Study power defines the ability of the study to demonstrate this association or causal relationship given that an association does actually exist. A more formal definition would be: the power of a statistical test is the probability that the test will reject a false null hypothesis (i.e. it will not make a type 2 error).
2. Yes. Eighty percent power is the lowest conventionally accepted level, giving an 80% chance of ending up with a p-value ≤ 0.05 (i.e. a statistically significant result) if there really is a difference.
3. In this paper, the null hypothesis is that providing free tea and coffee will make no difference to the LWBS rate.

   Type 1 error (α) = False positive. Falsely rejecting the null hypothesis when it is true, that is, getting a result that makes us think that free tea and coffee do make a difference when in reality they do not.

   Type 2 error (β) = False negative. Falsely accepting (technically *not rejecting*) the null hypothesis when it is wrong, that is, getting a result that makes us think tea and coffee do not make a difference when in reality they do.

Question 4

1. What is the difference between a primary and a secondary outcome measure? (1 mark)
2. What is the difference between qualitative and quantitative data? (1 mark)
3. In this study, are the secondary outcome measures quantitative or qualitative data? Explain your answer. (3 marks)

1. The end point is the result that you set out to look for. The main end point that the researchers are looking for (and the end point that the trial is powered to look at) is termed the primary end point. In this study this would be the LWBS rate. Other end points that are collected but that are not the primary end point are termed secondary end points; in this study this would be time to treatment and satisfaction scores.
2. Quantitative data are where a numerical value can be given to the data and this can be either discrete (i.e. with the number of people in a club it can be only 3 or 4, not 3.5) or continuous, where it can be anywhere on a scale. Qualitative data (also called categorical data) are where there are a fixed number of defined categories into which data are organized and this can either be nominal (i.e. given a name), such as hair colour, or ordinal (i.e. where there is a rank to the categories), such as first, second and third places in a race.
3. In the paper there are two secondary outcome measures. The waiting times are a quantitative result as they are a numerical value (time); the patient satisfaction results are also quantitative as patients have been asked to rate their satisfaction on a scale (giving a numerical result for satisfaction).

Question 5

1. What does a p-value represent? (2 marks)
2. What is meant by CONSORT statement? (2 marks)

1. A p-value is the probability of obtaining a result at least as extreme as the one observed, assuming the null hypothesis is true (i.e. assuming there is no effect in the population). The lower the p-value, the less likely the result is under the assumption of the null hypothesis (i.e. the less likely the result is to have occurred by chance).

   $p < 0.05$ means that the probability of obtaining the result by chance was less than 1 in 20. By convention, a p-value of less than 0.05 is the accepted threshold for statistical significance and is the level at which the null hypothesis can be rejected.

   In this paper, the primary outcome had a p-value of 0.04, meaning it was a statistically significant result.

2. A CONSORT statement is an evidence-based minimum set of recommendations for reporting randomized controlled trials. It offers a standard way for authors to prepare reports of trial findings, facilitating their complete and transparent reporting, and aiding their critical appraisal and interpretation.

Question 6

The following table was produced from a follow-up study in different hospitals but run with identical methodology. Calculate the absolute risk reduction, the relative risk, the relative risk reduction and the number needed to treat. (5 marks)

	LWBS	Waited to Be Seen
Free Tea and Coffee	330	610
No Free Tea and Coffee	410	530

Control event ratio (CER) = 410/(410 + 530) = 410/940 = 0.44
Experimental event ratio (EER) = 330/(330 + 610) = 33/94 = 0.35
Absolute risk reduction = 0.44 – 0.35 = 0.09
Relative risk (RR) = 0.35/0.44 = 0.80
Relative risk reduction = 0.09/0.44 = 0.20
Number needed to treat = 1/ARR = 1/0.09 = 11

Question 7

Your chief executive has read this paper and tells you she wants you to use some of the ED budget to provide free tea and coffee in the waiting room. What will you say to her? (6 marks)

I would recommend to the chief executive that we should not be making this change at this point.

(Not all of the below would be required for all the marks.)

I have concerns about some aspects of the trial methodology and hence the internal validity of the trial (i.e. how well it was designed and run).

This was an unblinded study, and although given the type of trial it is not unreasonable that the patients and clinicians were not blinded, we might have expected those collecting the data to be blinded. This leads to an increased risk of bias.

Although the paper states that free tea and coffee were not available in the control group, it would have been valuable to know what refreshments were available to people waiting.

When looking at the results, there were statistically significantly more medical patients and fewer minor patients in the control group than the intervention group. This raises the possibility that there were important differences in the populations between the control and intervention group. This may be an unrecognized confounder and the difference in LWBS may be due to the differences in minor patients in the different groups, rather than tea and coffee availability.

The satisfaction scores were recorded retrospectively and it is unclear how the subset who were contacted were selected, suggesting the possibility of recall and reporter biases, respectively.

The authors describe a 'significant' Hartland score change as 1 point, but their results show a difference of only 0.4 – highlighting the difference between statistical and clinical significance.

The external validity of the trial (i.e. how much I can generalize these results to the patients of other EDs) concerns me. This is a single trial run across only four hospitals in one part of the United Kingdom, and it was run over 2 weeks in a summer period (which incidentally coincided with the London Olympics), and therefore this population may not reflect the wider UK ED population.

Applicability: Finally, there is no mention of the cost of the intervention, making an assessment of its value difficult to judge. It is also unclear how centres restricted this from surgical patients who may not have been allowed to eat or drink prior to assessment. The treatment itself may have risks attached to it, which the authors have not discussed, such as delaying surgery.

Glossary

This list is not exhaustive but is representative of the key terms you need to have an understanding of when reading papers.

Absolute risk reduction: *See* risk.

Allocation concealment: The process whereby patients and researchers are unaware of which arm trial subjects will end up in once they have been enrolled in the trial. The important point is that if researchers or participants know what arm of a trial they are likely to go into, they may consciously or unconsciously change their decision about whether to enrol. Allocation concealment is the process where this is hidden until after enrolment and so reduces selection bias in a trial.

Alpha (α) value: α is the probability of making a type 1 error (a false positive – saying we reject the null hypothesis when in fact we should not). α is used in power calculations and is called the 'threshold of significance'. When considering a single test, if we set α at 0.05, we are saying that we are willing to accept a 5% chance of a false positive and that if the p-value we calculate comes under 0.05, we will accept the result as statistically significant.

Bayes' theorem: It is argued that this is the most important concept in medicine. There are lots of complicated explanations of the theorem in other books and on the Internet, but a simple way to explain it is to use an example. Essentially, the idea is that reaching a decision about how probable a diagnosis is relies on two stages. Assess the pre-test probability of someone having a diagnosis (e.g. your *clinical suspicion* whether a patient with chest pain is having a myocardial infarction [MI]) and then do a test to try to make the diagnosis. Any given test (e.g. in this case a troponin) will provide a likelihood ratio for the diagnosis – but this is a feature of the test and not the patient. Bayes' theorem states that the probability of the diagnosis is proportional to the product of the pre-test probability (in this case a feature of your history and diagnosis) and the likelihood ratio of the test. If your pre-test probability was low (e.g. a 19-year-old patient with muscular sounding pain after lifting weights) even with a raised troponin, the diagnosis of MI would be unlikely; if your pre-test probability was high (a 75-year-old arteriopath who smokes 80 cigarettes a day and has central crushing chest pain), a low troponin would not be sufficient to convince you he had not had an MI.

Bias: A systematic error in the way a trial is designed or run leading to inaccuracy in the result. There are many types of bias. When appraising a trial, one of the most important judgements to make is whether you think there was bias that might have affected the result. We have detailed various sorts of bias in the relevant chapters of the book, but the Cochrane Collaboration breaks down the areas that might have been affected by bias into the following steps:

1. *Selection of participants*: Was selection truly random and was allocation concealed before enrolment?
2. *Performance bias*: Were there any differences in the interventions (other than the treatment under investigation) given to the different trial groups that might have affected outcomes? Were all those involved in the trial adequately blinded to ensure that the different trial interventions were not known by those taking part in the trial or analyzing the results?
3. *Detection bias*: Were those assessing participant outcome adequately blinded to the intervention that the participants received?
4. *Attrition bias*: Do the authors adequately explain the reasons behind patients dropping out or being excluded from the study? Do their explanations seem reasonable?
5. *Reporting bias*: Question how the authors decided on what result they have chosen to report and whether it follows from the trial they originally designed.
6. *Anything else*: The above five areas are not exclusive, so also consider if there is anything else about the trial that would make you worried that the result had been influenced by bias.

Case control study: People with a disease are compared to those without the disease to find out what risk factors both groups have been exposed to in the past. It is therefore always retrospective. Pros: Quick and cheap; needs few participants; good for studying rare diseases or those where there is a long duration between exposure and outcome. Cons: Relies on recall and records to assess exposure; not good for looking at rare exposures; temporal relationships between exposure and outcome may be difficult to establish.

Causation and correlation: Correlation assesses the relationship between two variables, but it is an old adage of science that correlation does not prove causation.

In 1965, Sir Austin Bradford Hill presented a list of criteria by which we might judge a relationship to have causation rather than simply correlation. These have very much borne the test of time and are still used today:

1. *Strength*: The larger the association, the more likely causation exists.
2. *Consistency*: Repeated observations that confirm the link in different places, at different times, by different people.

3. *Specificity*: If the link is limited to specific situations, peoples and disease, then causation is more likely.
4. *Temporality*: Does the exposure to the variable always precede the development of the disease? This is particularly important in diseases where there may be a long time between development of the disease and diagnosis.
5. *Biological gradient*: Does a greater exposure to the variable (e.g. smoking more cigarettes) make one more likely to develop the disease?
6. *Plausibility*: Is there a biological rationale that is reasonable for why exposure to the variable might cause the disease?
7. *Coherence*: Does the evidence run in line with the other things known about the variable and the disease so far?
8. *Experiment*: If we intervene to reduce the exposure to the variable are we able to demonstrate a reduction in the disease or outcome?
9. *Analogy*: If the potential causation mirrors that seen in a similar exposure, we might be willing to accept less other evidence of causality.

Chance: A random variation that leads to imprecision in a study result.

Cohort study: Groups with and without an exposure are followed up to see how the development of an outcome differs between the groups. Pros: Good for resolving questions about aetiology, harm and prognosis; rare exposures; assesses temporal relationships and many outcomes; can give direct estimation of disease incidence rates. Cons: Not good for rare outcomes; can be expensive (e.g. long time from exposure to outcome); open to bias if people drop out. Cohort studies can be performed prospectively or retrospectively.

Confidence interval (CI): Gives a range of values that is likely to cover the true but unknown population value. CIs are more valuable than the p-value (primarily because of the difference between statistical significance and clinical relevance). CIs allow the reader to assess the likely clinical significance of where the result might lie. A CI can be given for various parameters: means, difference between means and ratios (RR, OR, etc.).

Confounding factor: A factor or variable within a study that is not part of the intervention and is not controlled for but which differs between the two groups being studied and which will affect the outcome of interest. Randomization is the tool we use to make sure that confounding factors (even those we do not know about) are equally spread between groups.

CONSORT diagram: A flow chart showing the flow of participants through each stage of a randomized trial.

CONSORT statement: The Consolidated Standards of Reporting Trials statement is a set of recommendations and tools intended to improve the way in which randomized controlled trials are reported and thus make them easier for readers to understand. It gives a suggested template depicting the passage of participants through a trial and shows what should appear in the various parts of the write-up (title, abstract, introduction, methods, results, discussion and other information).

Contingency table: A table used to show the results of diagnostic or therapeutic trials. In studies with two arms and two outcomes this is a 2×2 table and what we traditionally are used to working with.

In therapeutic trials, along the horizontal axis is the outcome and along the vertical axis, the intervention. In diagnostic studies, the gold standard is along the horizontal axis and the study under investigation along the vertical axis.

Controlled trial: People in the study are given one of two (or more) treatments or interventions.

Convenience sample: A type of non-probability sampling drawn from the part of the population that is close at hand; that is, a sample population is selected because it is readily available and convenient.

Crossover trial: All the people in the study receive one treatment and then halfway through the study crossover and receive the other treatment. Pros: Useful in studying rare diseases as subjects are their own controls. Cons: Difficulties with order effects, historical controls and carryover effects (e.g. if you give someone an analgesic and then they crossover to the placebo, the painkilling effect of the first drug may still be present; this can be avoided by using a sufficiently long 'wash-out' period between crossovers).

Cross-sectional study: Disease status and exposure status are measured simultaneously in a given population at a set time point. Pros: Good for establishing prevalence or establishing an association. Cons: Not good for establishing causation; recall bias is a problem; you need large groups; groups may be unequal sizes with an unequal distribution of confounders.

Data: Data can be described in various ways, as shown in Figure A.1.

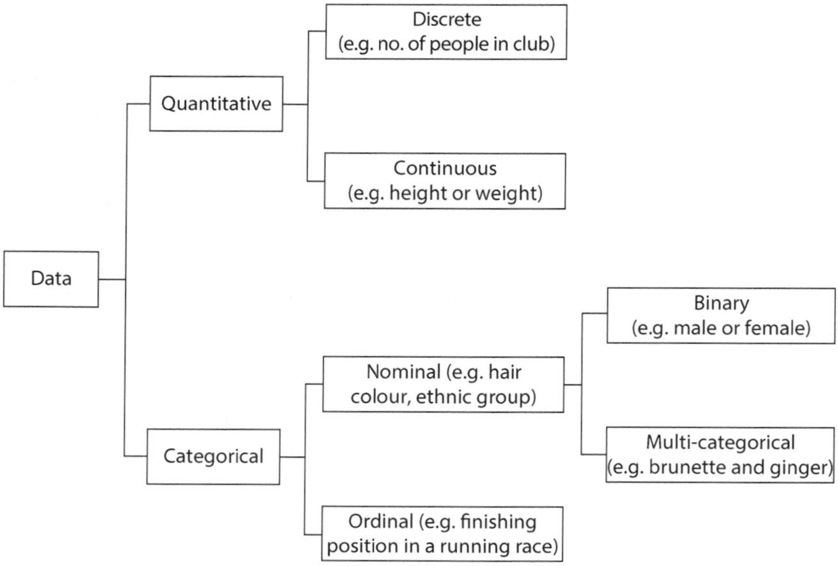

FIGURE A.1 Types of data.

Effectiveness: Does the intervention have the desired effect under ordinary circumstances? If external validity is present and the trial demonstrates an effect of the intervention, we can accept that a treatment has effectiveness.

Efficacy: Describes the impact of the intervention under optimal (trial) conditions. If internal validity is present and the trial demonstrates an effect, we can accept that a treatment has efficacy.

End points: The end point is the result that you set out to look for. The main end point that the researchers are looking for (and the end point that the trial is powered to look at) is termed the primary end point. It should be clearly stated at the start of the trial and the result of the primary end point should be easy to find in the results section. Other end points that are collected but that are not the primary end point are termed secondary end points, and it must be remembered that the trial has usually not been powered to look at them. A hefty degree of caution should be used when trying to draw conclusions from secondary end points. A further common way to divide end points is:

1. *Clinical end point*: An actual diagnosis of disease, symptom or sign. Death would perhaps be the best and most undeniable clinical end point.
2. *Surrogate end point*: A measure that may correlate with a real end point but is not necessarily guaranteed to. An example would be to measure gastric pH in an antacid trial rather than confirmed upper GI bleeding.

Error: (a) Type 1 error (α) = False positive. Falsely rejecting the null hypothesis when it is true. (b) Type 2 error (β) = False negative. Falsely accepting the null hypothesis when it is wrong.

External validity: The extent to which the results of a study can be extrapolated to a wider population. It is closely related to the term *generalizability*.

False negative: This is best explained using an example: when using a test, diagnosing someone as not having a disease when in fact they do have it.

False positive: This is best explained using an example: when using a test, diagnosing someone with a disease when in fact they do not have it.

Forest plot: A diagram produced in meta-analysis that shows the treatment effect from each trial and the overall treatment effect that has been calculated from the meta-analysis of the data. *See* Chapter 12.

Generalizability: Is the finding of the study applicable elsewhere?

Gold standard test: The best test available to diagnose a condition. It should be used as the comparison test in diagnostic studies looking at the ability of a novel test to detect the same disease.

Hawthorne effect: Considered to be the act of where observing a situation (including a clinical environment) improves the performance (and hence medical outcomes) of those *in all* groups within the trial. One conclusion of this is that the results obtained in research studies may be expected to be better than those that would be obtained in real life.

Hazard and hazard ratio: Hazard is a measure of how quickly an outcome occurs. If we are looking at death from myocardial infarction in an aspirin versus no-aspirin trial, we can calculate not only the overall death rate in each group but also the rate of death, and this is termed the hazard in each group. Although we like to keep things easy and we strongly recommend using risk and risk ratios when interpreting the results of an interventional trial, clearly there is value in an assessment that includes a measure of time to the outcome.

Hazard ratio is simply the hazard in the intervention group divided by the hazard in the control group. It is not the same as risk ratio and tells us how many participants in the intervention group will have the outcome compared with the control group at the next time point. It assumes that the hazard ratio remains constant between the two groups over time and should always be quoted alongside a time frame.

Incidence: The rate of occurrence of new cases over a given time, in a defined population.

Incidence = Number of new cases over a time period/Population size

Intention-to-treat analysis: All the study participants are included in the analysis as part of the group to which they are allocated, regardless of whether they completed the study, or received the treatment to which they were allocated. Intention to treat generally signifies a higher-quality study methodology and acts to reduce attrition bias.

Internal validity: The extent to which the methodology of the paper permits a reflection of the truth. That is, was the study methodologically good enough to demonstrate what was actually going on?

Inter-quartile range (IQR): A measure of spread or dispersion of a data set. It is the difference between the upper (75th) and lower (25th) quartiles and thus contains the middle 50% of the sample. It is smaller than the range and thus less affected by outliers. IQR (along with median) is used to describe data instead of standard deviation (and mean) when the data are not normally distributed, ordinal or from a small sample.

Note: Quartiles are values that divide sample data into four equal numbers of observations.

Jadad score: One example of a scoring system to assess the methodological quality of a trial – usually a randomized controlled trial.

Three questions:

1. Was the study described as randomized? (1 point)
2. Was the study described as double blind? (1 point)
3. Was there a description of withdrawals and dropouts? (1 point)

Two additional points if:

1. The method of randomization was described in the paper and was appropriate. (1 point)
2. The method of blinding was described in the paper and was appropriate. (1 point)

Points are deducted if:

1. The randomization was described but inappropriate.
2. The blinding was described but was inappropriate.

Kaplan–Meier curves: A widely used form of graph used to compare survival over time between groups in an interventional trial. It uses a method that incorporates the facts that not all participants will reach the end of the trial (through dropout or death) or indeed have the outcome of interest during the time frame of the trial. Instead of simply calculating event rates at various times, the event rate is adjusted for loss of participants (called 'censoring'). The curves that are produced for the different groups in the trial can be compared to see if there is a difference in outcome over time. Although widely referred to as 'survival curves', they can in fact be used to look at any binary outcome measure (death, acute myocardial infarction, relapse, discharge from hospital, etc.).

Kappa value: The Kappa statistic indicates the level of agreement between measurements made by different raters and gives an indication as to whether this agreement is more than can be expected by chance. It is also used to assess the level of agreement when the same observer does repeated observations with a test. Kappa is used for measuring categorical data – for our purposes, generally a 'disease present' or 'disease-free' answer.

The Kappa value lies between 0 and 1.0, where 0 is chance agreement and 1.0 is perfect agreement.

Agreement	Chance	Poor	Moderate	Substantial	Perfect
Kappa	0	0.20	0.40–0.60	0.80	1.0

Likelihood ratio (LR): Useful when considering an individual's test result in combination with your clinical findings. *See also* 2 × 2 table.

Mean: The sum of the values divided by the number of values. Normally distributed data is usually described using mean and standard deviation.

Median: The middle number of a group when they are ranked in order. The mean of the two middle values is taken if there is an even number of values. It is useful for skewed data and has the advantage of reducing the importance of outliers. Non-normally distributed (or non-Gaussian) data is usually described using median and inter-quartile range.

Minimization: A form of adaptive randomization. A running total is kept of all the levels of the prognostic factors of interest. The first patient in the trial is randomly allocated, but all subsequent patients are randomized using randomization weighted towards which assignment would minimize the imbalance.

Mode: The most frequently occurring value in a list. It has the advantage in that it can be used with non-numerical data (e.g. colours of cars).

Negative predictive value (NPV): The proportion of people with a negative test who do not have the disease. *See* 2 × 2 table.

Nominal data: A type of categorical data where the order of the categories is not important, for example, country of birth.

Normal data: Data that is normally (i.e. bell-shaped) distributed about the mean. Also known as Gaussian data.

Null hypothesis: This is the statement that therapeutic trials start with. The investigators will have a hypothesis that, for example, a drug lowers blood pressure. However, for the purpose of statistical inference, the researchers say that they are sampling from a population where the null hypothesis is true; that is, we are sampling from a population in which the intervention has no effect. The results of the trial are then used to either reject or not reject this hypothesis.

Number needed to treat (or harm): The number of people who need to be treated to achieve one outcome of interest. It is a powerful way to describe the value of an intervention. Mathematically it is 1 ÷ Absolute risk reduction. *See* risk.

Odds: Odds are a way of describing risk.

Mathematical odds = Desired events ÷ Undesired events

Odds ratio = Odds in treated group ÷ Odds in control group

Open trial: Both the researchers and participants know what treatments are being given to individuals. It is the opposite of a blinded trial.

Ordinal data: Data that can be ranked (put in order) or have a rating scale attached to it. You can count and order, but not measure, ordinal data, for example, first, second and third in a race.

Paired or unpaired data: Paired data are data for the same individuals at different time points – for our purposes, usually before and after an intervention. Unpaired data are two groups having different members (also known as 'independent data') as when we compare an interventional and control group in a randomized controlled trial.

Parametric statistics: Inferential methods that rely on the data following the normal distribution.

Per-protocol analysis: Also called 'on-treatment analysis'. Only those who sufficiently complied with treatment (as per the trial protocol) are included in the statistical analysis. It is a good way to demonstrate the actual effect of an intervention on people who take it (or can tolerate it) as the researchers intended, but it does not allow the reader to see how applicable the treatment is to the whole population.

Positive predictive value (PPV): The proportion of people with a positive test who have the disease. *See* 2 × 2 table.

Power: The power of a study defines its ability to demonstrate an association or causal relationship between two variables, given that an association exists, that is, when there is a relationship, the ability of the study to actually show it. A more formal definition would be: the power of a statistical test is the probability that the test will reject a false null hypothesis (i.e. it will not make a type 2 error).

If α has been set at 5% and the study powered to 80% (which is the lowest conventionally accepted level), then the study has an 80% chance of ending up with a p-value ≤ 0.05 (i.e. a statistically significant result) if there really is a difference.

Power = 1 – β, where β is the probability of a false negative (type 2 error). Four factors that affect the power of a study (and so should be mentioned in the methods of a paper):

1. α-value (set before starting – usually 0.05)
2. Sample size (therefore a power calculation should be done to calculate this before the trial starts)
3. Variability in data
4. Minimum clinically relevant difference/estimation of likely difference

Pragmatic trial: Pragmatic trials assess whether an intervention works under real-life conditions. It is simply concerned with whether an intervention works, not how or why.

All the people in a clinical setting (e.g. an outpatient clinic) are randomized to receive a particular treatment protocol. Pros: More reflective of clinical practice. Cons: More difficult to control; difficult to blind; difficulties with excessive dropout.

Prevalence: Point prevalence is the proportion of a defined population with a disease at any one time. Period prevalence is the proportion of a defined population with a disease during a given time period. Lifetime prevalence is the proportion of a population that has or has had a disease at a given time.

Prognostic factor: A prognostic factor is a variable which affects prognosis once you have the disease. Note the difference between this and a risk factor, which is a variable which affects the likelihood of getting the disease. For example, smoking is a risk factor for lung disease but not a prognostic factor. However, renal failure is not a risk factor for getting lung disease but is a prognostic factor in the chance of survival of the patient.

p-Value: A formal definition of a p-value can be given as: A p-value is the probability of obtaining a result at least as extreme as the one observed, assuming the null hypothesis is true (i.e. assuming there is no effect in the population). The lower the p-value, the less likely the result is under the assumption of the null hypothesis (i.e. the less likely the result is to have occurred by chance).

For many people, that is a bit of a mouthful and so we prefer: $p < 0.05$ means that the probability of obtaining the result by chance was less than 1 in 20. By convention, a p-value of less than 0.05 is the accepted threshold for statistical significance and is the level at which the null hypothesis can be rejected.

Calculation of the p-value is beyond the scope of this book.

Randomization: The process whereby an individual has an equal chance of entering any group within a study. Randomization reduces bias by distributing characteristics of patients that may influence outcomes (confounders – known and unknown) randomly between the groups.

Receiver operator characteristic (ROC) curve: Figure A.2 is used to assess diagnostic tests whereby the cutoff point for a positive and a negative test has been varied and then the specificity and sensitivity calculated for each cutoff. It is a tool that can be used to assess the best cutoff value for the test.

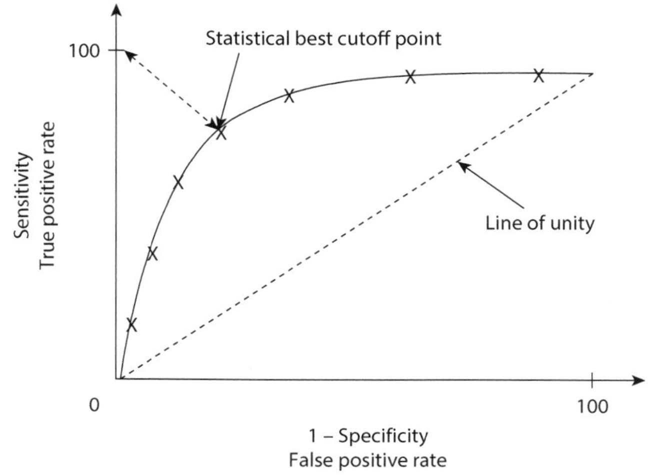

FIGURE A.2 Receiver operation characteristic curve.

The area under the curve (AOC) is a measure of how good the test is: 1.0 is perfect; 0.5 is no better than chance and the line would lie along the line of unity.

Statistically, the optimum cutoff point for a test (i.e. the balance between sensitivity and specificity) is where the line is closest to the top left corner of the graph; however, clinically we may choose a different point.

Regression analysis: Regression is a statistical method for looking at the relationship between one or more variables and outcomes. Consider a study measuring people's height and weight. If we were to plot the two on a graph, we might find that in general as height increases, so does weight. If the points lie approximately in a straight line, we can say there is a linear relationship between the two; if not there may be no relationship or there may be a non-linear relationship (e.g. the points lie in a curved shaped). The exact way this is done is beyond the scope of this book but a general understanding is valuable.

Linear regression analysis is the statistical tool used to analyze the relationship between continuous (i.e. not categorical) data when there is a linear relationship between the two. If we are looking at one variable and one outcome, we use *simple* linear regression; if we want to look at more than one variable, we use *multivariate* linear regression.

Logistic regression analysis is used, as with multivariate linear regression, when we want to know the effect of multiple variables on categorical data (e.g. dead or alive). If necessary, it is possible to convert a continuous outcome (e.g. D-dimer result) into a categorical outcome (e.g. positive or negative), but this must be done in a clinically appropriate way. Unlike in linear regression, the relationship between the variables and the outcome does not need to be linear.

Risk (statistics from a therapeutic paper): In clinical research, Risk = Probability.

Risk = Number of times an event occurs/Total possible events

Using a 2 × 2 contingency table, we can calculate the following:

	Outcome +ve	Outcome –ve
Experimental Group	a	b
Control Group	c	d

Risk in the control group = Control event rate (CER)

$$= c/(c + d)$$

Risk in the experimental group = Experimental event rate (EER)

$$= a/(a + b)$$

From this you can then calculate:

Absolute risk reduction (ARR) is the difference in risk between the groups and is useful as it allows you to calculate the number needed to treat.

$$ARR = CER - EER$$

Relative risk (RR) is a ratio of the risk in each group.

$$RR = EER/CER$$

Relative risk reduction = (CER – EER)/CER = ARR/CER

Number needed to treat (harm) is the number of people who need to be given the treatment to generate one positive (or negative) outcome, that is, 1/ARR.

Sensitivity: The ability of a test to rule out a diagnosis (SnOut). It is the proportion of people with the disease who test positive. *See also* 2 × 2 table.

Specificity: The ability of a test to rule in a diagnosis (SpIn). It is the proportion of people without the disease who test negative. *See also* 2 × 2 table.

Statistical tests: There are a number of different types of statistical tests which can be used to analyze data and generate a p-value.

Study types: There are a number of different study types. These are shown in Figure A.3.

2 × 2 table (statistics from a diagnostic study): This is used in diagnostic studies to compare the studied test to a gold standard.

		Gold Standard/Have the Disease	
		Disease Positive	Disease Negative
Index Test	Positive	A	B
	Negative	C	D

		Gold Standard/Have the Disease	
		Disease Positive	Disease Negative
Index Test	Positive	True positive (TP)	False positive (FP)
	Negative	False negative (FN)	True negative (TN)

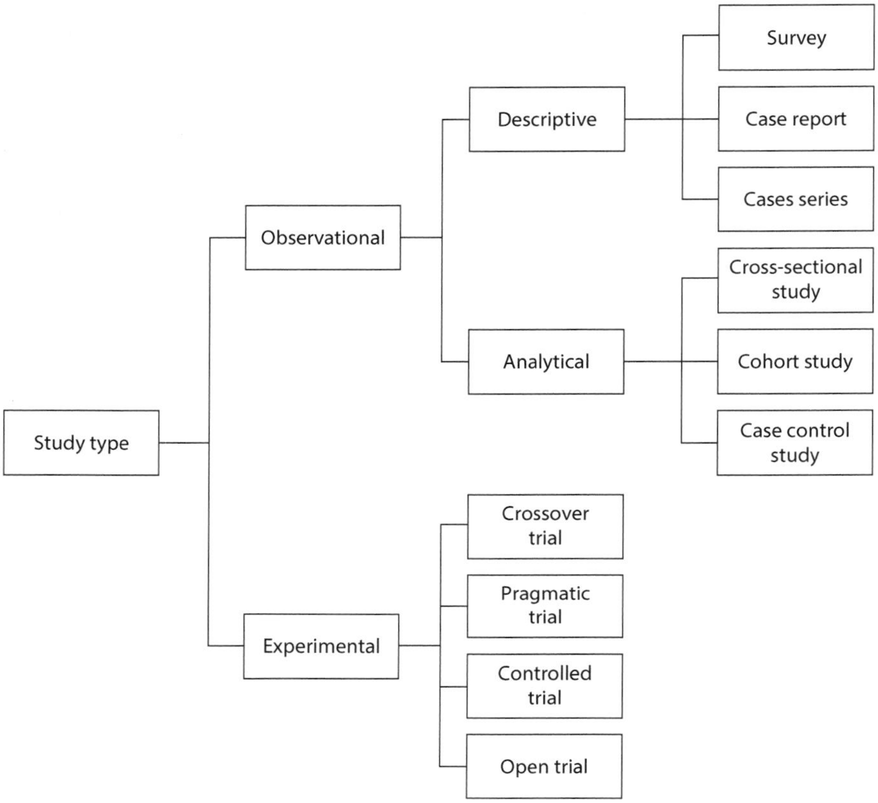

FIGURE A.3 Different study types.

The table then can be used to calculate a number of values:

Sensitivity = a/(a + c) = TP/(TP + FN)
= Proportion of people with the disease who test positive
= Sensitivity rules out (SnOut)

Specificity = d/(b + d) = TN/(FP + TN)
= Proportion of people without the disease who test negative
= Specificity rules in (SpIn)

Negative predictive value (NPV) = d/(c + d) = TN/(FN + TN)
= Proportion of people with a negative test who do not have the disease

Positive predictive value (PPV) = a/(a + b) = TP/(TP + FP)
= Proportion of people with a positive test who have the disease

Positive likelihood ratio (LR+) = Sensitivity/(1 – Specificity)
= Likelihood of someone with a positive result having the disease

Negative likelihood ratio (LR–) = (1 – Sensitivity)/Specificity
= Likelihood of someone with a negative result having the disease

Validity: Are the findings of the study true? *See* internal validity and external validity.

Index

A

Absolute risk reduction (ARR), 85
Adaptive randomization, 75
Alpha, 37
Alternative hypothesis, 33
Analysis of variance, 24
AOC, *see* Area under the curve
Appraising papers, approach to, 9–18
  abstract, 10
  authors and institution, 16
  bias, 15–17
  diagnostic purity bias, 11
  discussion and conclusions, 15
  financial interests, 18
  intervention and comparison, 13
  introduction, 10
  methods, 10–14
  other factors to consider, 15–18
  outcome measures, 13–14
  population, 11–12
  publishing journal, 18
  questions, 9
  references, 18
  results, 14–16
  take-home message, 18
  time, 14
  title, 10
  validity, 15
Area under the curve (AOC), 108
Attention bias, 77
Audit cycle, 139–140

B

Bayesian theory, 47, 51
Bell-shaped distribution of data, 23, 24
'Best available' evidence-based clinical environment, creation of, 137–142
  audit cycle, 139–140
  implementing new clinical practices, 137–139
  research, 140–141
  take-home message, 142
Bias, 15–17
  attention, 77
  definition of, 15
  diagnostic purity, 11
  in diagnostic studies, 93
  expectation, 77
  means of combating, 16
  specific to diagnostic studies, 93
  types, 16, 17
Blinding, 77–78, 93
Block randomization, 75

C

Case control studies
  design, 57
  methodology, 61–62
  odds in, 47
  results, 64
Categorical data, 21
CER, *see* Control event rate
CIs, *see* Confidence intervals
Clinical end points, 80
Clinical topic review (CTR), writing of, 129–132
  clinical question, 129–130
  critically appraising the papers, 131–132
  literature review, 130–131
  search engines, 130
Cluster randomization, 75, 83
Cohort studies
  design, 57–59
  methodology, 62–63
  results, 64
Coin toss, 43, 45
Composite end point, 80
Confidence intervals (CIs), 30
  95%, 32, 35
  p-values versus, 36
  take-home message, 42
Confounding, 80–82
Consolidated Standards of Reporting Trials (CONSORT), 9, 79
Contingency table, 84
Control event rate (CER), 44, 85
Correlation coefficient, 41
Cost–consequences studies, 120
Cost minimization studies, 119
Critical appraisal exams, approach to, 145–151
  design and methodology, questions about, 150
  diagnostic papers, 148–149
  exam technique, 145–146
  interpretation of paper, questions about, 151
  limitations of paper, questions about, 151
  meta-analysis, 149
  results, statistics, and 2 × 2 tables (questions about), 150–151
  take-home message, 151

therapeutic papers, 147
writing a summary, 146–149
Cross-sectional studies
methodology, 63–64
results, 64–65
studies, 59–60
CTR, *see* Clinical topic review (CTR), writing of

D

Data dredging, 39
Data types and moving from samples to populations, 21–32
categorical data, 21
data types, 21–22
epidemiological data, 22
example, 28
inferences about the whole population from sampled data, 28–32
Nerd's Corner, 26, 30
quantitative data, 21, 23–27
standard deviation, calculation of, 27
symbols, meaning of, 27
take-home message, 32
variance, calculation of, 27
Diagnostic papers, 91–102
biases, 93
blinding, 93
checklist, 111–112
design and methodology features, 91–95
example, 98, 101
high-risk man, 102
index test, 91
inter-observer reliability, 94
likelihood ratios, 99–100
low-risk man, 103
negative predictive value, 97
Nerd's Corner, 99, 102
nomogram, 104, 105
patient selection, 91–92
positive predictive value, 97
reference standard, 92–93
results, how to use and interpret, 95–102
test qualities, 94–95
writing a summary, 148–149
Diagnostic purity bias, 11
Dice, roll of, 43, 45

E

EBM, *see* Evidence-based medicine
Ecological studies
design, 60
methodology, 63–64
results, 64–65
Economic studies, 119–121
cost–benefit studies, 119
cost–consequences studies, 120
cost-effectiveness studies, 120
cost minimization studies, 119
quality-adjusted life years, 120
take-home points, 120
EER, *see* Experimental event rate
Eligibility criteria, 124
Epidemiological data, 22
Error, 36–37, 39, 40
Ethics, in qualitative research, 70–71
Ethnography, 69
Evidence, grades of, 6–8
ranking the strength of recommendation, 7
ranking the types of study, 7
take-home message, 8
Evidence-based medicine (EBM), 3, 138; *see also* 'Best available' evidence-based clinical environment, creation of
Exams, critical appraisal, *see* Critical appraisal exams, approach to
Expectation bias, 77
Experimental event rate (EER), 43, 85
Experimental studies, 5
External validity, 15, 55

F

Forest plot, 125
Free Open Access Medical Education (FOAM), 137
Funnel plots, 124

G

Gaussian distribution of data, 23, 24
Glossary, 183–195
Gold standard (diagnostic papers), 92–93
Google/Google Scholar search, 131
Grounded theory, 69

H

Hawthorne effect, 84, 140
Heterogeneity, 125
Hypothesis
alternative, 33
null, 33
study, 33
testing, 33–34

I

Index test, 91
Intention-to-treat analysis, 82
Internal validity, 15, 55
Inter-observer reliability, 94
Introduction, methods, results and discussion (IMRaD) format, 10, 123

J

Journal club operation, 133–135
choosing articles, 134
critical appraisal of articles, 135
presentation, 135
setup, 133–134
take-home message, 135

K

Kaplan–Meier curves, 115
Kappa value, 94, 109, 124
Kendall's correlation, 41

L

Likelihood ratios (diagnostic papers), 99–100
'Lived experience,' 69

M

MCID, *see* Minimum clinically important difference
Meta-analysis, 123–126
abstraction of data, 124
analysis, 125
checklist, 126
eligibility criteria, 124
forest plot, 125
funnel plots, 124
heterogeneity, 125
Kappa value, 124
literature search, 123–124
odds in, 47
purpose of, 123
review articles, types of, 123
selection of papers, 124
systematic review, 123
take-home message, 126
writing, 123–125
writing a summary, 149
Minimum clinically important difference (MCID), 38

N

National Institute for Health and Care Excellence (NICE), 8, 131, 139
Nerd's Corner, 21
accuracy of sample mean, 30
converting probabilities to odds and vice versa, 49
descriptions of variance of data, 26
diagnostic papers, 99, 102
95% confidence intervals, 35
odds in case control studies, 47
odds in meta-analysis, 47
odds ratios appearing to exaggerate claims, 46
probabilities, 39, 44
prognostic papers, 113
screening papers, 110
NICE, *see* National Institute for Health and Care Excellence
Nomogram, 104, 105
Normal distribution, value of, 28–29
Null hypothesis, 33
Number needed to treat (NNT), 85, 86

O

Observational studies, 55–66
case control studies, 57
cohort studies, 57–59
conclusions, 65
cross-sectional studies, 59–60
design, 56–60
ecological studies, 60
internal versus external validity, 55
methodology, 60–64
recognition of observational study, 55
researcher questions, 56
results, 64–65
take-home message, 66
use of appropriate trial, 56
Odds, 44–45
calculating post-test probabilities using, 47–49
coin toss, 45
dice, roll of, 45
having superior mathematical properties, 47
probability versus (risk), 45–47
ratios appearing to exaggerate claims, 46
in therapeutic trials, 45
Open trial, 77

P

Papers, types of, 3–7
environment, 4
experimental studies, 5, 6
observational studies, 7
questions, 3–4
researcher intervention, 5
results, 5
take-home message, 8
ways to label a trial, 4
Parametric tests, 24
Patient assessment team (PAT), 83
Pearson's correlation, 41
Per-protocol analysis, 82
Phenomenology, 69
Placebo effect, 73
Populations, moving from samples to, *see* Data types and moving from samples to populations

Power calculation, 38, 42
Practice papers, 153–181
answers, 162–166, 177–181
competing interests, 156
conclusion, 156, 172
data analysis, 154
discussion, 155–156, 171–172
introduction, 153, 167
journal article, 167–181
methods, 153–154, 167–168
questions, 158–161, 173–176
results, 154–155, 168–169
Primary end point, 80, 179
Probability, 43–51
calculating post-test probabilities using odds, 47
coin toss, 43
control event rate, 44
converting post-test odds to probabilities, 49
converting probabilities to odds and vice versa, 49
dice, roll of, 43
experimental event rate, 43
Nerd's Corner, 39, 44, 46, 49
odds, 44–45
odds versus probability (risk), 45–47
pre-test probability, 50
risk versus probability, 43–44
take-home message, 51
Prognostic papers, 113–117
checklist, 117
definitions, 113
methods, 113–115
morbidity, 115
mortality, 115
Nerd's Corner, 113
prognostic factors, 114–115
results, 115–116
study participants, 113–114
survival curve, 115, 116
take-home message, 116
p-value, 34, 36, 81

Q

QALY, *see* Quality-adjusted life years
Qualitative data, 21, 23–27
average value, 23
distribution of the data, 23–25
measures of spread and location, 26
normal distribution, 23
parametric tests, 24
skewed data, 25
statistical tests, 24
Qualitative papers, 67–72
appraisal of, 71
definition of qualitative research, 67
ethics in qualitative research, 70–71
ethnography, 69
examples, 67, 68
grounded theory, 69
methodologies, 69
mixing methods, 69
need for qualitative research, 67–68
phenomenology, 69
take-home message, 72
types of qualitative research, 68–70
Quality-adjusted life years (QALY), 120
Quasi-randomization, 75

R

Randomization, 75
Randomized controlled trials (RCTs), 3, 113
Randomized control trials, design and methodology features of, 73–82
accounting for patients, 78–79
allocation of trial participants and randomization, 74–76
analysis of results, 82
blinding, 77–78
clinical end points, 80
comparison against another intervention, 73–74
confounding, 80–82
intention-to-treat analysis, 82
interventional trials, 81
outcome, 79–80
per-protocol analysis, 82
placebo effect, 73
selection of trial participants, 74
surrogate end points, 80
Receiver operating characteristic (ROC) curve, 107–108
Regression, 42
Relative risk reduction, 86
Results section (therapeutic trial), interpretation of, 84–90
absolute risk reduction, 85
calculations, 85–89
contingency table, 84
example, 86–88
number needed to treat, 86
odds ratios, 88
relative risk, 86
relative risk reduction, 86
Review articles, types of, 123
Risk, 45–47
factor, definition of, 113
Nerd's Corner, 46
ratio, 46
trial, 45, 46
ROC curve, *see* Receiver operating characteristic curve

S

Screening papers, 109–112
- considerations, 109
- example, 109
- gold standard way of telling the impact of screening test, 109
- Nerd's Corner, 110
- take-home message, 111

SD, *see* Standard deviation
Secondary end point, 80, 179
SEM, *see* Standard error of the mean
Service delivery therapeutic trials, 83–84
Significance, definition of, 33
Simple randomization, 75
Skewed data, 25
Spearman's rank correlation, 41
Standard deviation (SD), 27, 28
Standard error of the mean (SEM), 30, 31
Statistical power, 37–38
Statistical significance, threshold for, 37
Statistical tests, types of, 24, 40–42
Statistics used in papers, 33–42
- alternative hypothesis, 33
- clinical significance of the result, 33
- confidence intervals, 35
- data dredging, 39
- definition of significance, 33
- error, 36–37
- errors in studies, looking out for, 38–40
- hypothesis testing, 33–34
- Nerd's Corner, 35, 39
- null hypothesis, 33
- p-values, 34
- statistically significant result, 33
- statistical power, 37–38
- statistical tests, types of, 40–42
- take-home message, 42
- threshold for statistical significance, 37

Stratified block randomization, 75
Study hypothesis, 33
Surrogate end points, 80
Symbols, meaning of, 27
Systematic reviews, 123, 129

T

Take-home message
- approach to appraising papers, 18
- 'best available' evidence-based clinical environment, creation of, 142
- confidence intervals, 42
- critical appraisal exams, approach to, 151
- economic studies, 120
- grades of evidence, 8
- journal club operation, 135
- meta-analysis, 126
- observational studies, 66
- odds and probability, 51
- prognostic papers, 116
- qualitative papers, 72
- screening papers, 111
- standard deviation, calculation of, 32
- therapeutic papers, 89
- types of papers, 8

Therapeutic papers, 73–90
- absolute risk reduction, 85
- checklist, 90
- number needed to treat, 85
- open trial, 77
- randomized control trials, design and methodology features of, 73–82
- results section, interpretation of, 84–90
- service delivery therapeutic trials, 83–84
- take-home message, 89
- writing a summary, 147

Threshold for statistical significance, 37
t-tests, 24
Type 1 error, 36–37, 39
Type 2 error, 37, 40

V

Validity, 15, 55
Variance, calculation of, 27

W

Well's score, 100
Whole population, inferences about (from sampled data), 28–32
- accuracy of sample mean, 29–31
- making predictions about populations from a single sample, 30
- standard error of the mean, calculation of, 31
- why normal distribution is valuable, 28–29